Essentials of Experimental Pharmacology

Volume 1

General Concepts

Essentials of
Experimental Pharmacology
Volume 1
General Concepts

Sunil B. Bothara

M. Pharm, Ph.D.

Professor and Principal

C.U. Shah College of Pharmacy and Research

Wadhwan City

Dist. Surendranagar

Gujarat.

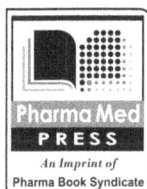

PharmaMed Press

An imprint of Pharma Book Syndicate

A unit of **BSP Books Pvt., Ltd.**

4-4-309/316, Giriraj Lane,

Sultan Bazar, Hyderabad - 500 095.

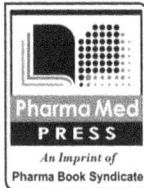

Published by

PharmaMed Press
An imprint of Pharma Book Syndicate
A unit of BSP Books Pvt., Ltd.

4-4-309/316, Giriraj Lane, Sultan Bazar, Hyderabad - 500 095.
Phone: 040-23445605, 23445688; Fax: 91+40-23445611
E-mail: info@pharmamedpress.com

ISBN : 978-93-52300-59-4 (HB)

Dedicated to

My Parents
Shri. Bhikchand Jain & Mrs. Suraj Jain
and

my two Pharmacology teachers
Prof. (Dr.) R. Balaraman, my Ph. D. guide
and
Dr. Sanjay B Kasture
who taught me during UG + PG
for their invaluable contribution in my life

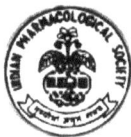

Indian Pharmacological Society
President

Prof. Ramesh K. Goyal
M.Sc. (Medical), Ph.D. (Pharmacy)
F.I.C., FAMS, FICN, FIPS, FIACS, FNASc
Vice-Chancellor

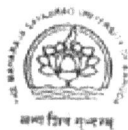

The Maharaja Sayajirao University of Baroda

Office University Road, Fatehgunj, Vadodara 390002 Gujarat India

Foreword

Pharmacology is one of the fastest changing subjects in pharmacy and medical sciences. Within a century there have been 4 revolutions: Chemotherapeutic (before 1940), biological (1940-70), molecular (1970-1990) and genomic (2000 and beyond) revolution. Similar revolution have occurred in experimental pharmacology from whole animal (upto 1950) to isolated tissue experiments (1950-1980), use of cell based assays (1980-2000) to transgenic animals and micro arrays (2000 and beyond).

Although in developing countries like India, pharmacology could not keep pace with this developing science there has been a change in attitude towards experimental pharmacology. One of such change has been a restricted use of animals and application of computer assisted learning. For this purpose CPCSEA regulatory has came into force and through AICTE and PCI, all colleges and universities in India have been instructed for replacement of some of the experiments with computer assisted learning.

The book written by Dr Sunil Bothra is probably the first of its kind, such that it gives information about not only CPCSEA but also computer aided learning, keeping routine experiments in place. I am sure this book will serve a good guide for the students of pharmacy and medical colleges. I compliment and congratulate Dr. Sunil Bothra for bringing out such a book.

(Ramesh K. Goyal)

Preface

It is a great pleasure, indeed, to present this book to budding Pharmacologists and their teachers from Pharmacy, Medical and Veterinary streams studying either at Undergraduate level or Postgraduate level. All must be aware of the fact that Pharmacology is the soul of the Drug Discovery, Therapeutics and Toxicology like branches that are vital for the mankind to get rid of various diseases with either avoidance of adverse effects or information about adverse effects.

Pharmacology is studied to know the actions and effect of various agents on biological systems, may it be cells, tissues or whole animal. Experimental Pharmacology is the primary step to make the students familiar with experiments that can be reinforcing their theoretical knowledge of the subject that can be extrapolated to screen newer compounds for their future prospects during drug discovery programme. Therefore, it becomes very important to study the subject with a perspective to study it with basics. In the present book series I have tried to make separate issues covering General Considerations, *in vivo* and *in vitro* experiments so as to make it easy and convenient to students, teachers and librarians.

As stated above Pharmacology is extremely important subject for present and future activities relevant to drug discovery and usage. Therefore, it is prudent to know and strengthen our basics before actually starting for experimental part. The first book of the series i. e. General Considerations is aimed to have the topics which must be learned well before actual experimentation.

The first Chapter – Introduction will deal with brief information of Pharmacology-what is it? Why to have experiments in Pharmacology and what basics we must know? Animal usage is integrated part of Pharmacology. At the same time there are genuine concerns about rational and humane use of animals including efforts to minimize the usage of animals along with animal housekeeping. In India we have a regulatory authority for the same named Committee for the Purpose of Control and Supervision of Experiments on Animals (CPCSEA). During my long tenure in academics, I came to know that many institutes still find it difficult to get CPCSEA approval due to unawareness on CPCSEA guidelines and therefore finding difficult to conduct experiments. The chapter on 'Regulatory Aspect' and the 'Appendices' should help the beginners. Since the present alternatives are not enough to replace use of animals, the use of animals has become essentiality. It becomes most important to plan the studies in such a way to reduce the animal usage as much as possible to avoid loss of precious lives of animals without substantial cause. There are many ways suggested to rationalize animal usage and are briefly known as 3 R's. The use of computers (softwares) is also proving highly beneficial to implement these 3R principles. The efforts are being made to introduce this new and highly exciting area for the benefit of all the enthusiastic learners of Pharmacology. The Pharmacy Council of India (PCI) has directed the colleges to minimise the use of animal experiments and make maximum use of Computer Assisted Learning (CAL). The Chapter on CAL will help to implement the directives by PCI. Despite of all the efforts it will not be possible to replace animals totally from the Pharmacology experiments and therefore substantial information on various laboratory animals and their characteristics to be studied before designing experiments. It will also be important to know various techniques to handle the animals, to administer various agents through different routes of administration and withdrawal of various fluids etc. The instruments and equipments also form an important component of experimental Pharmacology. Many sophisticated instruments are fortunately made available with great abilities to provide minute details and better recording facilities, in addition to applications of computerised algorithms. Yet the challenge to Pharmacologists is big one as comparatively lesser new molecules and targets are discovered in last 2 decades. I expect more enthusiasm and wish all the aspirants best in their endeavour. I am proposing to provide optimum details for the learners in various facets of experimental pharmacology and therefore an introductory session on Statistics was inevitable.

I believe that my efforts to reproduce the knowledge, as graced by my erudite teachers, in appropriate and in lucid manner will be accepted nicely by the readers. It is my humble request to all the lovers of Pharmacology to write their critical comments about this book to the author so that future editions can be improved.

Bothara Sunil B.

botharasb1@gmail.com

Acknowledgements

I am sincerely thankful to Dr. R. Raveendran, Professor of Pharmacology, JIPMER, and creator of important softwares like ExPharm EP-Dog etc., for permitting to provide details of his softwares and also sharing his knowledge about sources available for the same. I am highly indebted to **Prof. (Dr.) R.K. Goyal Sir,** Honourable Vice Chancellor, The M. S. University of Baroda and President, Indian Pharmacological Society for his magnanimity in writing Foreword to this book. No words can thank him for his kind gesture. I am grateful to Prof. Sainath Iyer, Postgraduate Professor in Pharmacology (PG), C U Shah Medical College, Surendranagar; for his painstaking efforts in critical editing of this book. His guidance backed by few decades experience and expertise in Pharmacology was of immense help in improvement of this book. I am thankful to my colleagues Mr. R. Murugan, Lecturer in Pharmacology & an excellent painter for the sketches in this book and Mr. Santosh Vaidya for the help. It is not easy to pursue such endeavour when your personal computer showing signs of no cooperation with recurrent problems. My staff member Mr. Narendra who helped to solve problems in my PC and spared his PC for some time. Thanks are due to him.

This project would not have taken off without vision of Shri. Anil Shah, Director / Proprietor Pharma Book Syndicate, Hyderabad who envisaged having a book on experimental pharmacology for his publishing house from me. I profusely thank him for his faith and whole hearted efforts for successful publication of this book. Thanks are also due to his staff members, particularly Mr. Naresh, Mrs. P. Kalpana. I must give special thanks to Mr. Niraj Ranjan, Gujarat Marketing representative, who was instrumental in initiating the process, for his management and creating consistent pressure on me to complete the book in time.

As always rock solid backing from my wife Mrs.Rachana and two sons Master Ayush and Master Navkaar could enable me to concentrate on this project. The two younger chaps even forgo their rights on computer till the completion of project. Their contribution is immense and it is beyond thanks.

- Author

Contents

1

Introduction

Pharmacology is a branch of biology which deals with study of Drug. There are several branches viz- Pharmacokinetics dealing with study of Absorption, Distribution, Metabolism and excretion of drugs (What body does to Drug), Pharmacodynamics dealing with study of actions and effects of drug (What drug does to body), Toxicology deals with study of toxic effects of drugs and treatment of poisons/toxicities, Experimental Pharmacology deals with study of various models and parameters to test the hypotheses related to either Pharmacokinetic /Pharmacodynamic /toxicologic characteristics of the given agent. The therapeutics (Pharmacotherapeutics) is also one branch dealing with study of applications of medicinal agents in therapeutic (treatment of diseases). Clinical Pharmacology is application of Pharmacology in Clinical Practice i.e. during treatment of patients (in Clinic).

This brief introduction of some important branches of Pharmacology underlines importance of experimental pharmacology, which forms base for study of various hypotheses and bring out some answers to contribute other branches of Pharmacology. The experimental Pharmacology can be broadly divided in two major types of study-

A. Preclinical studies and B. Clinical studies

A. *Preclinical studies:* The studies performed before clinical studies are the Preclinical studies. Since human beings can not be directly subjected to risk arising due to administration of new or unknown agent, studies must be conducted before going for human studies so as to get information about pharmacokinetic and pharmacodynamic aspects of new intervention. Thus preclinical studies involve experiments performed using any other living beings/things except human beings. These other living beings may be various experimental animals categorised as rodents/ non-rodents /primates/other animals or various cells obtained from different sources i.e., specific tissues from various animals and may also involve use of bacteria, viruses, protozoa, metazoan and other such unicellular or multicellular organisms used for performing preliminary studies to test activities of the given agent/s.

Thus preclinical studies involve a very broad field which utilizes biological sources other than human beings for acquiring information on many aspects like-

Broad Activities (Macro level)	**Specific Activities (Micro level)**
1. To understand physiologic/ pathophysiologic role of various biological agents like hormones, vitamins, enzymes, neuro-transmitters, ions, proteins and other biological elements etc. In Short it includes study of all cellular and extra cellular components of organism for understanding normal functioning and disease status of the organism.	1. To study and confirm role of these components using or setting appropriate models[1] and endpoints[2] / parameters[3]. 2. Application of these models and parameters in elucidating /confirming activity of given NCE[4]

---

[1] *Animal Model*- Inducing the human disease like situation (simulation) by using suitable method (may be induced by either one or more techniques like chemically, alteration of housekeeping, surgically or genetically altered physiology simulating the disease status in humans)

[2] *End Points*- The product studied in the animal model should demonstrate a beneficial effect analogous to the intended outcome in humans. Primary study endpoints, which should be specifically discussed with the review division, generally are the enhancement of survival or prevention of major morbidity in most of the studies. The dose response for these endpoints should be explored fully and established. Although secondary endpoints can provide useful information about the animal model and the activity of the product as studied in the animal model, ordinarily, only primary endpoints can serve as the basis of approval.

[3] *Parameters*- The data required to substantiate the effects of given agent e.g. blood sugar level, blood pressure, agonistic/antagonistic effects produced etc.

E.g., Diabetes can be induced in animal by various ways (Chemically using streptozotocin/ alloxan, surgically- by pancreactomy and diet induced) accordingly called as alloxan model of diabetes. End points can be Primary-survival with and without treatment and impact on complications. Secondary endpoints / Parameters can be blood glucose level, glycosylated haemoglobin level, insulin level, ketone bodies and other which can predict mechanism of action e.g. estimation of Glucose Transporters or potassium channel activity etc.

3. To study Pharmacokinetic characteristics i. e. absorption, distribution, metabolism and excretion of either such NCE[4] or existing drug where formulation process is altered. Particularly bioavailability[5] information is obtained using time vs. plasma concentration curves.

3. To confirm role played by various organs/ tissues/ cells/ enzymes/proteins etc. in these pharmacokinetic activities like active/passive absorption, protein binding, role of tissue/enzyme in metabolism with pathway/s, routes and

4. To study the Pharmacodynamic characteristics of the given substance i.e. Effects of drug either at *in vivo* or *in vitro* level

4. To know the mechanism of action at cellular or sub-cellular level for bringing out those effects.

5. To study the toxicological aspects of the intervention/drug i. e. effects other than desired/ expected and detrimental to body are observed using various toxicity testing activities like- acute, sub acute and chronic.

5. To study the mechanism of action at cellular or sub-cellular level producing this deleterious effects. To verify the short term and long term impact on all anatomical (histological) and physiological alterations leading to toxicity.

Clinical Studies: The studies performed using human subjects / volunteers are known as Clinical Studies. Clinical Studies involve clinical research and clinical trials.

At the core of the drug development process is a fundamental understanding of the clinical pharmacology of the drug substance. Clinical pharmacology can be thought of as a translational science in which basic information about the relationship between a drug's dose, local or systemic exposure and response (related to either efficacy or safety) is applied in the context of patient care. Knowledge of this relationship, which is a key to

---

[4] *NCE- New Chemical Entities:* New Chemical Entity- According to the U.S. Food and Drug Administration, a new chemical entity (NCE) (also known as new molecular entity (NME)) is a drug that contains no active moiety that has been approved by FDA in any other application (Molecule not recognized as Drug). is a chemical molecule developed by the innovator company in the early drug discovery stage, which after undergoing clinical trials could translate into a drug

[5] *Bioavailability:* Rate (per unit time) (quantity) by which the drug reaches systemic circulation after administering it extra-vascularly (other than directly in blood vessel). It gives both – Rates applied for ADME and quantity (concentration) changing with respect to time.

successful therapeutics, and how it is altered by the intrinsic (age, gender, renal function, etc.) and extrinsic (diet, drugs, life-style) factors of an individual patient is one of the major contributions of clinical pharmacology to drug development and regulatory decision-making.

Once a lead compound with the intended pharmacological action is identified, the step-wise process to characterize and potentially optimize its pharmacokinetic (PK) properties (i.e., absorption, distribution, metabolism, and excretion), as well as to minimize its pharmacokinetic limitations (e.g., poor absorption), begins in humans as part of phase I human clinical trials. Soon after, other principles of clinical pharmacology [e.g., pharmacokinetic-pharmacodynamic (PD) relationships] become critical to the evaluation and selection of the most appropriate dosing regimen of the drug in a carefully selected target population enrolled in phase II clinical trials. These trials form the scientific rationale for subsequent dose selection in large-scale phase III clinical trials where the primary goal is to provide adequate evidence of efficacy and relative safety of the drug. Phase III trials are the most expensive and time-consuming component of the overall drug development process and many believe that paying careful attention to doing clinical pharmacology "homework" has the greatest potential to reduce the failure rate of new drugs at this near final stage of development.

Often, in parallel with phase III clinical trials, a group of clinical pharmacology studies, such as those in special populations, are conducted in human volunteers to develop a knowledge database of factors influencing drug exposure. These data are crucial for an understanding of when, and how much, to adjust dosage regimens. Because these studies typically focus on changes in systemic exposure, as a surrogate marker for either efficacy or toxicity, the availability and the intelligent use of exposure (e.g., dose, PK measurements)-response (e.g., biomarkers, surrogate clinical endpoints, clinical outcomes, PD) relationships to interpret the results of these studies become critical to information for various sections of the product label.

These studies can be broadly classified into two broad categories: 1. those dealing with patient-intrinsic factors that include gender, age, race, diseases states (primarily renal and/or hepatic impairment), and genetic (e.g., activity of cytochrome P450 enzymes) factors, and 2. those dealing with patient extrinsic factors that include drug-, herbal- and nutrient-drug interactions, environmental variables (e.g., smoking, diet), and lifestyle factors.

Clinical Research: The NIH definition of clinical research is based on the 1997 Report of the NIH Director's Panel on Clinical Research that defines clinical research in the following three parts: 1. Patient-oriented research. Research conducted with human subjects (or on material of human origin such as tissues, specimens and cognitive phenomena) for which an investigator (or colleague) directly interacts with human subjects. Excluded from this definition are in vitro studies that utilize human tissues that cannot be linked to a living individual. Patient-oriented research includes: (a) mechanisms of human disease, (b) therapeutic interventions, (c) clinical trials, or (d) development of new technologies. 2. Epidemiologic and behavioural studies, 3. Outcomes research and health services research.

Clinical Trial: a clinical trial is operationally defined as a prospective biomedical or behavioural research study of human subjects that is designed to answer specific questions about biomedical or behavioural interventions (drugs, treatments, devices, or new ways of using known drugs, treatments, or devices).

As per the revised Schedule 'Y' of the Drugs & Cosmetic Act (2005), "a clinical trial is a systematic study of new drug(s) in human subject to generate data for discovering and/or verifying the clinical, pharmacological (including pharmacodynamic, and pharmacokinetics), and/or adverse effects with the objective of determining the safety and/or efficacy of the new drugs". Clinical trial of drugs is a randomised single or double blind controlled study in human participants, designed to evaluate prospectively the safety and effectiveness of new drugs/ new formulations. The new drug as defined under the Drugs and Cosmetic Rules 1945 (DCR), and subsequent amendments include:

(i)   a new chemical entity (NCE);

(ii) a drug which has been approved for a certain indication, by a certain route, in a certain dosage regimen, but which is now proposed to be used for another indication, by another route, or in another dosage regimen;

(iii) a combination of two or more drugs which, although approved individually, are proposed to be combined for the first time in a fixed dose combination (FDC).

Clinical trials are used to determine whether new biomedical or behavioural interventions are safe, efficacious and effective. Clinical trials of experimental drug, treatment, device or behavioural intervention may proceed through four phases:

Phase I Clinical Trial: **Human Pharmacology-** These are done to test a new biomedical or behavioural intervention in a small group of people (e.g. 20-80) for the first time to explore activities, PK and evaluate safety (e.g. To determine a safe dosage range, and identify side effects). These trails are conducted to- Assess tolerance, Define/describe PK and PD, Explore drug metabolism and drug interactions, Estimate activity. E.g. Dose-tolerance studies, Single and multiple dose PK and/or PD studies, Drug interaction studies.

Phase II Clinical Trial: **Therapeutic Exploratory-** These are done to study the biomedical or behavioural intervention in a larger group of people (several hundred) to determine efficacy and to further evaluate its safety. These trails are conducted so as to explore use for the targeted indication, estimate dosage for subsequent studies, provide basis for confirmatory study design, endpoints, and methodologies. E.g. Earliest trials of relatively short duration in well- defined narrow patient populations, using surrogate or pharmacological endpoints or clinical measures, Dose-response exploration studies.

Phase III Clinical Trial: **Therapeutic Confirmatory-** These are done to study the efficacy of the biomedical or behavioural intervention in large groups of human subjects (from several hundred to several thousand) by comparing the intervention to other standard or experimental interventions as well as to monitor adverse effects, and to collect information that will allow the intervention to be used safely. These trails are conducted to demonstrate /confirm efficacy, Establish safety profile, Provide an adequate basis for assessing the benefit/risk relationship to support licensing, establish dose-response relationship. E.g. Adequate and well controlled studies to establish efficacy, randomised parallel dose response studies, clinical safety studies, studies of mortality/ morbidity outcomes, large sample trials, and comparative studies.

NIH-Defined Phase III Clinical Trial: **Therapeutic Use-** For the purpose of the Guidelines on the Inclusion of Women and Minorities, an NIH-defined Phase III clinical trial is a broadly based prospective NIH-defined Phase III clinical investigation, usually involving several hundred or more human subjects, for the purpose of evaluating an experimental intervention in comparison with a standard or control intervention or comparing two or more existing treatments. Often the aim of such investigation is to provide evidence leading to a scientific basis for consideration of a change in health policy or standard of care. The definition includes pharmacologic, non-pharmacologic, and behavioural interventions given for disease prevention, prophylaxis, diagnosis, or therapy. Community trials and other population-based intervention trials are also included.

Phase IV Clinical Trial: **(POST-MARKETING SURVEILLANCE):** **Therapeutic Use-** studies are done after the intervention has been marketed. These studies are designed to monitor effectiveness of the approved intervention in the general population and to collect information about any adverse effects associated with widespread use. Because of genetic diversity among humans, it is possible that a new drug will cause adverse effects in only a small group of genetically similar people, which may not have been apparent during clinical trials. As the new drug is given to more and more people, careful monitoring is necessary to avoid this possibility. Drugs are taken off the market if post-marketing surveillance reveals previously undetected side effects. This phase of clinical trails is conducted to refine understanding of benefit/risk relationship in general or special populations and/or environments, identify less common adverse reactions, and refine dosing recommendation. E.g. Comparative effectiveness studies, studies of mortality/morbidity Outcomes, studies of additional endpoints, large sample trials, pharmacoeconomic studies

Clinical testing is complex and time-consuming, averaging 14 years to complete Phase I through III testing to gain FDA approval. Sometimes, drugs will fail in clinical tests because the animal tests did not accurately predict their effects in humans. Often people wonder why it takes so long to develop a new drug and why sometimes a drug treatment is not found to be dangerous until after it is sold to the public.

2

Understanding Basics

Before starting experiments it is important to know various basics covering Pharmacology with respect to basic pharmacology, drug-receptor interactions, quantitative and qualitative aspects of drug actions. Further, it is also important to learn basics, terminology and methods for making solutions of various concentrations.

Receptor: A cellular macromolecule, or an assembly of macromolecules, that is concerned directly and specifically in chemical signalling between and within cells. Combination of a hormone, neurotransmitter, drug, or intracellular messenger with its receptor(s) initiates a change in cell function. Several types of receptors may be identified: peripheral membrane proteins, many hormone and neurotransmitter receptors are transmembrane proteins i.e. transmembrane receptors are embedded in the phospholipid bilayer of cell membranes which allow the activation of signal transduction pathways in response to the activation by the binding molecule called as ligand and Metabotropic receptors are coupled to G proteins and affect the cell indirectly through enzymes which control ion channels.

Ionotropic receptors (also known as ligand-gated ion channels) contain a central pore which opens in response to the binding of ligand.

Another major class of receptors is intracellular proteins such as those for steroid and intracrine peptide hormone receptors. These receptors often can enter the cell nucleus and modulate gene expression in response to the activation by the ligand.

Ligand: A molecule which binds to a receptor is called a "ligand," and may be a peptide (such as a neurotransmitter), a hormone, a pharmaceutical drug, or a toxin, and when such binding occurs, the receptor goes into a conformational change which ordinarily initiates a cellular response. Ligand-induced changes in receptors result in physiological changes which constitute the biological activity of the ligands. Ligand may be agonist or antagonist.

Receptor reserve: There is said to be a receptor reserve (also known as spare receptors) for that particular agonist in that particular tissue. This was speculated after it was found that despite of blocking receptors with irreversible antagonist (making no receptor available for agonist), the agonist could exhibit the action. It is believed that there is no receptor reserve for a drug which acts as a partial agonist in the tissue. The receptor reserve may vary between tissues, depending on the number of receptors in the particular tissue and the efficiency of coupling between them and their effector mechanism. Consequently, a partial agonist in one tissue may appear to act as a full agonist in a tissue with a higher receptor reserve

2-State Receptor Concept: It is also believed that many receptors exist in 2 states –Active and inactive state. Full agonist can convert maximum receptors in active state while partial agonist does it partially. The agonist prevents activation of receptor by agonist.

Orphan Receptor: The receptors which are identified and the binding of ligand is also known but their **Effector Mechanism** (see below second messenger) / effects are not elucidated.

Species homologue (or species variant): A receptor for a particular neurotransmitter which mediates the same physiological function in two species and is found in similar tissue locations. The two receptors differ in amino-acid sequence to a small degree (approx. 10% or less), giving rise to differences in the affinity of some antagonists or the relative potencies of agonists

Subtype: Subtypes of receptor are those which, in a single species, are activated by the same family of endogenous ligands but exhibit sufficient differences in their pharmacological properties or molecular structure to justify being classified separately. Traditionally, subtypes have been identified using drugs which can selectively activate them or antagonize the effects of agonists with markedly different potencies (the usual rule of thumb is that there should be at least a 10-fold difference in antagonist affinity, i.e. one log unit difference in pK_B value, when postulating the existence of a novel receptor subtype).

Second messenger: It is the intracellular substance (e.g. cyclic AMP or inositol phosphates) of which the concentration varies due to activation of membrane receptors and which in turn controls further intracellular events like protein phosphorylation, neurotransmitter release or membrane polarization etc. It is a key substance in **Effector Pathway** (several effector pathways are explained in chapter 3- Agonists and Antagonists) for eliciting a response of given receptor-ligand interaction.

Agonist: A drug which has ability to bind a receptor (affinity) and activate (intrinsic activity) it resulting in to some activity (response) at the site of action like contraction, relaxation, secretion, enzyme activation, etc which is called as pharmacological response.

Affinity: It means the ability of ligand to bind the receptor. Potency (described below) depends on affinity.

Intrinsic activity: A term devised by Ariens in 1954 to describe the mathematical relationship between receptor occupancy and tissue response i.e. ability of ligand (agonist only) to elicit the response. The term efficacy (explained below) is a measure of intrinsic activity.

Response: In simplest form it means the measurable changes brought by the ligand which could be almost anything. For example, the response might be enzyme activity, accumulation of an intracellular second messenger, membrane potential, secretion of a hormone, heart rate or contraction of a muscle.

Partial agonist: An agonist which, no matter how high a concentration is applied is unable to produce maximal activation of the receptors. Indicating that has less intrinsic activity than full agonist.

Antagonist: A drug has ability to reduce the effect of an agonist when concomitantly administered or expected to attenuate activity of agonist physiologically present. This is possible because the agent has affinity towards receptor but it lacks the intrinsic activity. It is classified as follows-

Competitive Antagonism: The agonist and antagonist compete for the same binding site or combine with adjacent sites that overlap (syntopic interaction). A third possibility is that different sites are involved but that they influence the receptor macromolecule in such a way that agonist and antagonist molecules cannot be bound at the same time. The effects of a competitive antagonist may be overcome by increasing the concentration of agonist, thereby shifting the equilibrium and increasing the proportion of receptors which the agonist occupies.

Reversible (surmountable) Competitive antagonism: If the agonist and antagonist form only short-lasting combinations with the receptor, so that equilibrium between agonist, antagonist, and receptors is reached during the presence of the agonist, the antagonism will be surmountable over a wide range of concentrations (*reversible competitive antagonism*).

Irreversible Competitive antagonism (Insurmountable or unsurmountable competitive antagonism: Some antagonists, when in close enough proximity to their binding site, may form a stable covalent bond with receptor (*irreversible competitive antagonism*), and the antagonism becomes *insurmountable.* It is said that no spare receptors remain available for action of agonist making it impossible to elicit the response.

Non-Competitive Antagonism: Agonist and antagonist can be bound to the receptor simultaneously; antagonist binding reduces or prevents the action of the agonist with or without any effect on the binding of the agonist. There are many mechanisms are believed to play- allosteric changes in receptor making it either inactive, inaccessible to the agonist or by modulating the receptor site negatively.

Reversible (surmountable) Non-Competitive antagonism: If the binding is not covalent i.e. the change made in receptor is transient and can be easily overcome by addition of more agonist; the antagonism is called as reversible non competitive antagonism. Here the addition of agonist shifts the activity towards positive impact by reducing the negative impact of antagonist on receptor (i.e. negative modulation).

Irreversible Non-Competitive antagonism (Insurmountable or unsurmountable Non-competitive antagonism: If the binding is covalent or the changes made in receptor are irreversible as there won't be activity even by addition of more agonist, the antagonism is called as irreversible non-competitive antagonism. The receptor is permanently modified so that the negative modulation caused by it can not be restored to normalcy.

Functional antagonism (physiological antagonism): Truly speaking, they are not antagonists as per our above definitions but are agonists having exactly opposite effects to each other. The receptor, mechanism of action may differ but the final effect shall be opposite.

Inverse agonist: A drug which produces an effect opposite to that of an agonist, yet acts at the same receptor. The best established example is Flumazenil that acts at the benzodiazepine receptor. Such compounds have also been described as **negative antagonists**, or as having **negative efficacy**.

Specificity: Relative potency of a drug between the receptors for two different endogenous ligands (e.g. chlorpromazine is specific for D_2 dopamine receptors as compared to other receptors like α, H_1 etc).

Selectivity: Relative potency of a drug between two receptor subtypes for the same endogenous ligand. This is a relative rather than absolute term that should always be quantified (e.g. prazosin is 30-fold selective for α_1-adrenoceptors relative to α_1-adrenoceptors).

EC_{50}: It is the molar concentration of an agonist which produces 50% of the maximum possible response for that agonist. Other percentage values (EC_{25}, EC_{40}, etc) are sometimes used.

IC_{50}: Where an agonist causes an inhibitory response, the IC_{50} is the molar concentration which produces 50% of its maximum possible inhibition.

Potency: A measure of the concentrations of a drug at which it is effective. Lower is a concentration producing desired response higher is a potency of given ligand. For agonists, EC_{50}, IC_{50}, K_A or pD_2 are usually used, while pA_2, K_B or pK_B are used for antagonists.

Relative potency: The ratio of the potency of a test drug (i.e. its EC_{50}, IC_{50}, etc.) to that of a standard drug.

Efficacy: A term introduced by Stephenson to describe the way in which agonists vary in the response they produce even when they occupy the same number of receptors. It is ability of an agonist to produce maximal response (irrespective to dose). High-efficacy agonists can produce their maximal response while occupying a relatively low proportion of receptors; agonists of lower efficacy cannot activate the receptors to the same degree and may not be able to produce the same maximal response even when they occupy the entire receptor population, thereby behaving as partial agonists

Relative efficacy: Stephenson proposed a numerical definition of agonist efficacy in which a pure antagonist (i.e. one totally devoid of any agonist activity) was defined as having zero efficacy, and a drug with an efficacy of 1 would, by definition, produce a maximal response at full occupancy that was 50% of the maximal response to a high-efficacy agonist. A more practical method of comparing agonist efficacy is to determine relative efficacy, i.e. to compare the ratio of the receptor occupancy at which two agonists produce the same response. There is no upper limit on the numerical value of efficacy or relative efficacy.

Desensitization or Tachyphylaxis: A reduction in the response to an agonist while it is continuously present at the receptor, or a progressive reduction in the response upon repeated presentation of the agonist.

Quantitative Aspects in Pharmacology

After understanding the basic terminology in sequence of events, it will be interesting to know applications of same for quantitative estimations in Pharmacological experiments.

Dose-response curves (DRC)

As the name suggest Dose-response curves are plots of concentration (in different mathematical forms) versus response obtained to it. Usually, the term "dose-response curve" is more frequently used to describe *in vitro* experiments than *in vivo* experiments. Since between the binding of the agonist to a receptor and the production of the response many steps can occur, depending on which drug is used and which response is measured, dose-response curves can have almost any shape. In majority of times the log dose-response curves follow a standard shape known as Sigmoid Curve as shown below.

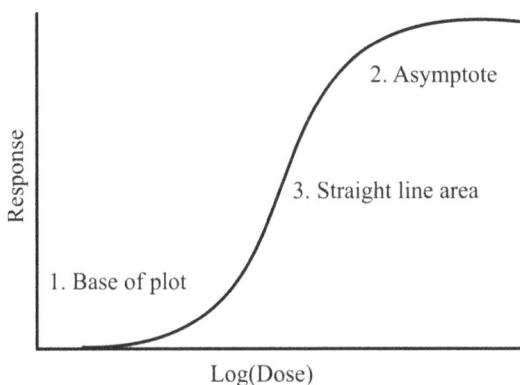

Log(Dose)

The log dose is selected or use of semi log paper is preferred so as to accommodate large range of values of several doses (usually 10-20) of agonist, approximately equally spaced on a logarithmic scale. Suppose dose is selected in the ascending order of 1, 3, 10, 30, 100, 300, 1000, 3000, and 10000 μM, which corresponds to their approximate log values: 0.0, 0.5, 1.0, 1.5, 2.0, 2.5, 3.0, 3.5, and 4.0 respectively, which are equally spaced and covering very big range of doses from 1 to 10,000 μM.

The response plotted on Y- axis may be taken in various forms like percent response of maximum response produced (where largest response being 100%), frequency of response (this is mostly applicable *in vivo* methods) in which number of times the response is obtained is counted, percent frequency (where sum total of all number of responses is made and considered as 100 %, the relative value of each individual response is compared accordingly).

There are 3 distinct features of a standard dose-response curve: 1. the baseline response (Bottom of curve)- which indicates relatively less activity may be due to activation of receptors, building equilibrium with the receptors etc, 2. the maximum response (Top of curve) which is also called as asymptote and related to saturation of receptors and slowly even spare receptors, 3.The middle straight line portion which indicate linear proportionate activity (response) with increase in drug concentration. This portion is useful in most of the pharmacological estimations involving DRC e.g. bioassay involving interpolation assays etc.

Uses of Log dose- percent response curve-

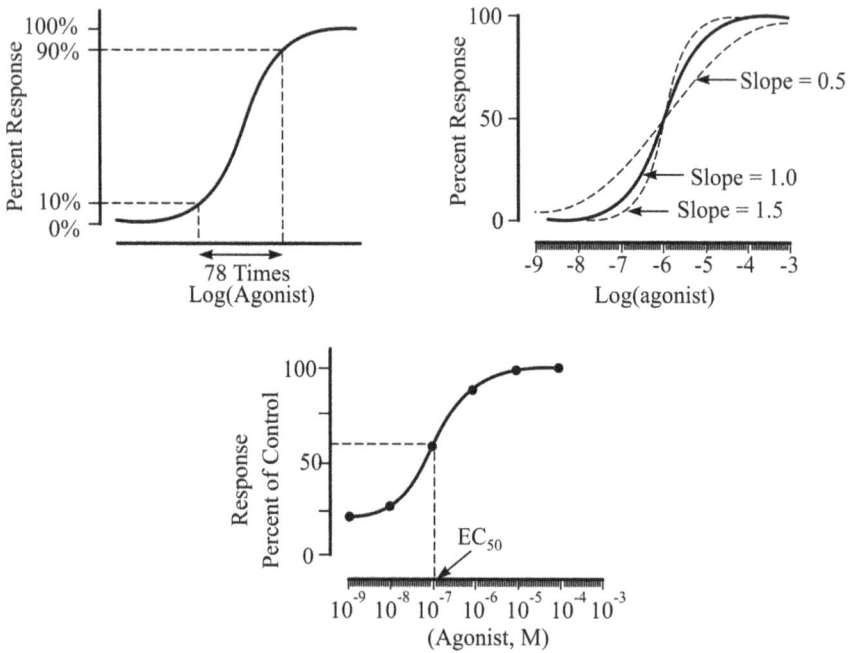

The Figures shown above explains various purposes these graphs can serve in experimental pharmacology. The details are explained below.

The steepness of a dose-response curve

The first from above figures shows that 78 times more agonist is needed to achieve mid 80% response than 10% response at both ends. This provides true dose-response linearity. The second figure shows that some dose-response curves are either steeper or shallower than the standard curve. The steepness is quantified by the Hill slope (slope factor). A dose-response curve with a standard slope has a Hill slope of 1.0. A steeper is curve higher will be the slope factor while a shallower curve will have a lower slope factor.

The EC_{50}

The third figure shows EC_{50} determination. We have already defined it in above section but to revise again- it is the concentration of agonist that provokes a response half way between the baseline (Bottom) and maximum response (Top). It means that until the baseline and maximum response are defined EC_{50} can not be obtained.

Dose-response curves in the presence of antagonists

Competitive surmountable antagonists: A dose-response curve of agonist performed in the presence of a fixed concentration of antagonist will be shifted to the right, with the same maximum response and (generally) the same shape.

Irreversible Competitive antagonism (Insurmountable or unsurmountable competitive antagonist: A dose-response curve performed in the presence of a fixed concentration of antagonist will not only be shifted to the right but also the reduction in maximum response and change in the shape.

In the figures given below the difference between competitive and non competitive antagonism is explained. The first figure compares effect of agonist and partial agonist. It can be observed that partial agonists can not reach to maxima. The second figure explains effect of competitive antagonist while the third figure shows change in response of agonist (line-1) due to either effect of 3 doses of competitive antagonist (line 2, 3, 4) or 3 doses of irreversible antagonist (line 5, 6, 7). It shows that even 10 times increase in concentration of reversible antagonist can elicit same response as an agonist except increase in dose of agonist. While irreversible antagonism can not produce same response again.

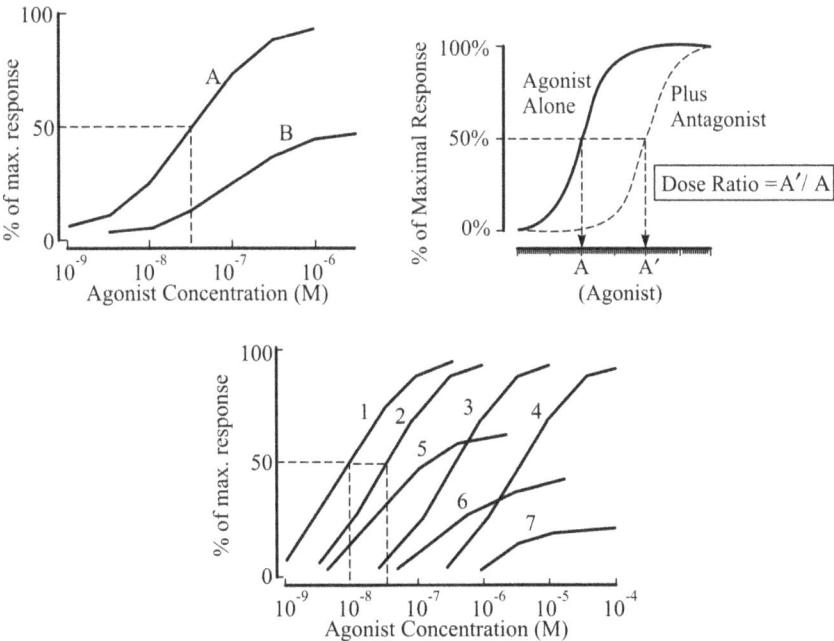

Limitations of dose-response curves

Fitting a sigmoidal (logistic) equation to a dose-response curve to determine EC_{50} (and perhaps slope factor) does not give all the details about an agonist. The observed EC_{50} is due to the agonist's *affinity* and intrinsic activity. There can be many possibilities-1.The agonist could bind with very high affinity, but have low efficacy once bound. 2. It could bind weakly with low affinity, but have very high efficacy. Thus two very different drugs could have the *same* EC_{50}s and maximal responses (in the same tissue).

(a) Other Important Definitions and Equations:

Concentration ratio or Dose-ratio

Concentration of agonist producing a defined response (usually but not necessarily 50% of maximum) in the presence of an antagonist, divided by the concentration producing the same response in the absence of antagonist. This gives measure of antagonist activity.

Kinetics of binding

The simplest assumption about the nature of the binding of drugs to receptors is that one molecule of drug (D) binds reversibly to one receptor molecule (R) to form a drug-receptor complex (DR):

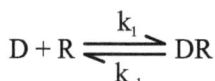

$$D + R \underset{k_{-1}}{\overset{k_1}{\rightleftharpoons}} DR$$

The rate of the forward reaction is equal to k_1 [D] [R], where k_1 is the association rate constant. (The square brackets signify the molar concentration of the terms they enclose). The rate of the reverse reaction equals k_{-1}[DR], where k_{-1} is the dissociation rate constant. At equilibrium, the rate of association equals the rate of dissociation, i.e.

$$k_1 \text{ [D] [R]} = k_{-1}\text{[DR]}$$

After rearranging,

$$\frac{k_{-1}}{k_1} = K_D = \frac{[D][R]}{[DR]}$$

K_D, the dissociation constant, may thus be defined either as the ratio of the dissociation and association rate constants, or as the concentration of drug which, at equilibrium, occupies 50% of the receptors (i.e. [DR] = [R], so K_D = [D]).

Occupancy

The activity is proportional to the number of receptor occupied and Occupancy is the proportion of receptors to which a drug is bound. It can be calculated from the Hill-Langmuir adsorption isotherm:

$$\text{Occupancy} = \frac{[D]}{K+[D]}$$

Where [D] is its concentration and k or K_D _ The dissociation constant for a drug determined by saturation analysis. The units are moles per litre, and it is the concentration of drug which, at equilibrium, occupies 50% of the receptors. Its reciprocal is called the affinity constant, sometimes abbreviated to K_{aff}.

Occupancy in presence of antagonist: Gaddum derived the equation that describes receptor occupancy by agonist in the presence of a competitive antagonist. Drug A is the agonist having molar concentration is [A] and dissociation constant Ka while drug B is the antagonist having molar concentration is [B] and dissociation constant is Kb. If the two drugs compete for the same receptors, fractional occupancy by agonist (f) equals:

$$f = \frac{[A]}{[A]+K_a\left(1+\dfrac{[B]}{Kb}\right)}$$

The presence of antagonist increases the EC_{50} by a factor equal to 1+ [B]/Kb. This is called the dose-ratio as shown above in figure 2 explaining shift of curve in presence of antagonist- If concentration A of agonist gives a certain response in the absence of antagonist, but concentration A' is needed to achieve the same response in the presence of a certain concentration of antagonist, then the dose-ratio equals A'/A. A different dose ratio will be obtained if different concentration of antagonist is used. If the two curves are parallel, the dose-ratio can be assessed at any point. It is better to calculate the dose-ratio at the EC_{50} in the presence of antagonist divided by the EC_{50} in the absence of antagonist. The above equation is of great help as there is no need to know what fraction of the receptors is occupied at the EC_{50} (and it doesn't have to be 50%).

Gaddum equation: It gives the value of **pK_B**- A measure of the potency of a competitive antagonist; the negative log of the molar concentration which at equilibrium would occupy 50% of the receptors in the absence of agonist, in the case as shown above in which a single concentration of antagonist has caused a parallel shift of the agonist concentration-response curve.

$$pk_B = \log(\text{conc.ratio} - 1) - \log(\text{antagonist conc.})$$

For a competitive antagonist (i.e. one where the slope of the Schild plot equals 1), the pK_B is theoretically equal to the pA_2 value. In practice, there may be some discrepancy. The pK_B value should also be equal to the pK_i value for the compound determined in a binding assay, although there may again be a discrepancy caused by the use of different media, etc.

Dissociation constant or K_B: The dissociation equilibrium constant for a competitive antagonist; the concentration which would occupy 50% of the receptors at equilibrium. The reciprocal of K_B is called the **affinity constant** or the **association constant**.

Schild Method

Arunlakshana and Schild showed the method for the calculation of the potency of competitive antagonists. It assumes that any particular level of response is associated with a unique degree of occupation and activation of the receptors by the agonist. It is also based on other assumptions and criteria like - (i) the agonist and antagonist act at a single receptor type; (ii) the binding of both agonist and antagonist is competitive and reversible; (iii) responses are measured when both agonist and antagonist are at equilibrium with the receptors and (iv) the antagonist causes parallel rightward shifts of the log agonist concentration-response curve with no change in the maximum response.

If the antagonist is competitive, the dose ratio equals one plus the ratio of the concentration of antagonist divided by its Kd for the receptor. (The dissociation constant of the antagonist is sometimes called Kb and sometimes called Kd)

$$\text{Dose ratio} = 1 + \frac{[B]}{K_b} = 1 + \frac{[Antagonist]}{K_d}$$

A simple rearrangement gives **Schild equation** and the logarithmic transformation of this equation is given above as the Gaddum equation.

$$\text{Dose ratio} - 1 = \frac{[Antagonist]}{K_d}$$

$$\log(\text{dose ratio} - 1) = \log([Antagonist]) - \log(K_d)$$

Schild plot: Thus when experiments with several concentrations of antagonist are performed and a graph is plotted with log (antagonist) on the X-axis and log (dose ratio -1) on the Y-axis. If the agonist and antagonist are competitive, the Schild plot will have a slope of 1.0 and the X and Y-intercept will equal the logarithm of the Kd of the antagonist. If the X-axis of a Schild plot is plotted as log (molar concentration), then the intercept multiplied with minus one gives the value called the pA_2 (p for logarithm, like pH; A for antagonist; 2 for the dose ratio when the concentration of antagonist equals the pA_2). The pA_2 (derived from functional experiments) will equal the Kd from binding experiments if antagonist and agonist compete for binding to a single class of receptor sites. The **Schild slope** gives information about the nature of the antagonism. The slope of a Schild plot should equal 1 if all of the assumptions made above are correct. If the slope increase than 1, it indicates less action of antagonist (positive co-operativity) which may be due either the binding of the antagonist, depletion of a potent antagonist from the medium by receptor binding or non-specific binding (e.g. to glassware or partitioning into lipid), or lack of antagonist equilibrium. As the slope becomes lesser than 1 may indicate more action of antagonist (negative co-operativity) which may be due to either increase in the binding or removal of agonist by a saturable uptake process or it may arise because the agonist is acting at a second receptor type. In last situation may result in curved Schild plots. Many other reasons may also play roles in variation of slopes from the theoretical value.

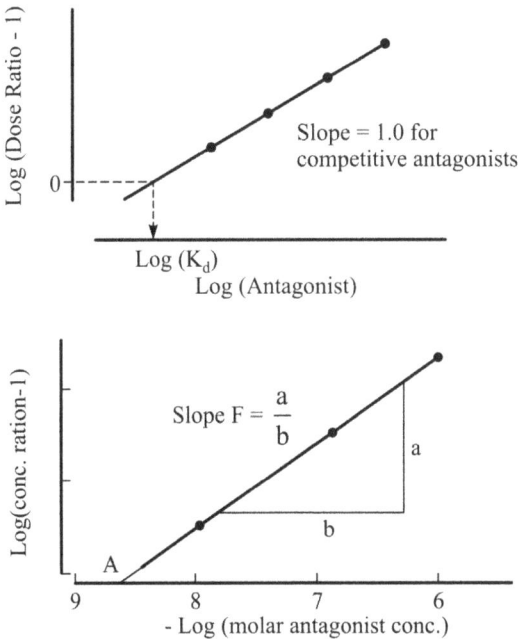

Schild plot- Derived by plotting log (concentration ratio - 1) on the y axis against the negative log of the molar concentration of antagonist on the x axis. The **pA₂** value for the antagonist is given by intercept (A). The slope F=a/b is explained in text.

Furchgott analysis: It is a method of measuring the affinity of an agonist by comparing its concentration-response curve before and after inactivating a proportion of the receptors with an irreversible antagonist.

pD$_2$: The negative logarithm of the EC_{50} or IC_{50} value is called as **pD$_2$** value and it is indicative of efficacy of the agonist.

pA$_2$: This is the logarithmic measure of the potency of an antagonist; the negative log of the concentration of antagonist which would produce a 2-fold shift in the concentration-response curve for an agonist. It is calculated by extrapolating the line on a Schild plot to zero on the y-axis.

Solutions in Experimental Pharmacology

Physiological Salt Solution (PSS)

It was accidentally observed by Ringer that presence of salt solution increased the duration of experiment. It led to discovery of various physiological salt solutions suitable for different tissues obtained from variety of animal species. The basic composition of PSS is made in such a way that it will provide necessary electrolytes to maintain electrolyte balance, osmotic balance and glucose is added for synthesis of energy. The table below gives composition of various PSS used for *in vitro* experiments.

Constituent	Frog Ringer	Krebs'	Tyrode	Ringer-Locke	De Jalen	Artificial CSF**
NaCl	65g	69g	80g	90g	90g	72.5g
KCl	1.4g	3.5g	2.0g	4.2g	4.2g	1.4g
$MgSO_{(4)}.7H_{(2)}O$	--	2.9g	2.6g	--	--	4.9g
$NaH_{(2)}PO_{(4)}.2H_{(2)}O$	0.65g	--	0.65g	--	--	--
$KH_{(2)}PO_{(4)}$	--	1.6g	--	--	--	1.75g
Glucose	20g	20g	10g	10g	5g	19.8g
$NaHCO_{(3)}$	4g	21g	10g	5g	5g	21g
1.0M $CaCl_{(2)}$	10.8ml	25.2ml*	18ml	10.8ml	2.7ml	2ml

Constituent	Role in PSS
Sodium Chloride	Provide Na^+ and Cl^- ions which are essential for excitability, maintenance of ionic equilibrium and osmotic pressure
Potassium Chloride	Provide K^+ ions and Cl^- ions which are essential for excitability, maintenance of ionic equilibrium and osmotic pressure
Magnesium Sulphate	Counter act Ca^{++} activity, Helps in reducing spontaneous activities.
Sodium Dihydrogen	Phosphate Buffer- helps in pH maintenance, Provide Na^+ ions, Phosphate ions and osmotic pressure

Contd....

Phosphate	
Potassium Dihydrogen Phosphate	Phosphate Buffer- helps in pH maintenance, Provide K^+ ions, Phosphate ions and osmotic pressure
Glucose	Source of energy (ATP) by oxidative pathway and osmotic pressure
Sodium Bicarbonate	Buffering agent for alkaline pH. Provide Na^+ ions, Carbonate ions and osmotic pressure
Calcium Chloride	Source of Ca^{++} ions essential for contraction and other physiological role.

Important aspects

1. *Temperature:* The temperature should be maintained as per requirement of the experiment to be performed which is usually 37^0C in most of the experiments. The details of temperature maintenance are mentioned in chapter 10 (instruments). Increased temperature may lead to early tissue damage due to fatigue while if the temperature is reduced it may lead to smaller, inadequate responses.

2. *pH:* The temperature should be maintained as per requirement of the experiment to be performed which is usually 7.2-7.4 in most of the experiments. Usually the components of PSS can automatically give desired pH. However it is must to confirm the same before start of experiment and set it using dilute acid (HCl) or base ($NaHCO_3$). During experiments too pH changes due to metabolism by the tissue. Use of carbogen (mixture of 95 %O_2 and 5% CO_2) recommended in many preparation to avoid such change in pH.

3. *Preparation of Solutions:* It is must to use demineralised distilled water for making the solutions. The best way is to prepare concentrated stock solutions of each component, except glucose, of required PSS and mixed in such a way that solutions of highly soluble substances are mixed first and at the end stock solutions of least soluble substances are added to avoid precipitation of substance like calcium salts. Other way is to weigh the required quantity of each ingredient for 10 and 5 litres solution and mix the same in the order mentioned above. Approximately 90 % of final volume is made and pH is confirmed, it is to be adjusted if it deviates from the required range and the final volume is made. Add glucose just before dispensing for use so that the already made solution can be used in next instance if precipitate is not formed. After adding glucose the solution must be finished in one day. Unused PSS and the solution remaining in organ bath assembly must be discarded to avoid microbial (mostly fungal) growth in it spoiling the container and assembly.

4. While making modified PSS as required for certain experimental condition the care must be taken that the tonicity (osmotic pressure) of PSS is maintained.

Making Drug Solutions

Many factors play role in making drug solutions-

1. Solubility of drug- The information can be obtained from Pharmacopoeias or standard book like Merck index which gives solubility of drug. The terms used by Indian Pharmacopoeia (IP) to describe solubility at 20 to 30 ^{0}C are-

Descriptive term	Approx volume of solvent in ml/gm of solute	Descriptive term	Approx volume of solvent in ml/gm of solute
very soluble	less than 1	sparingly soluble	from 30 to 100
freely soluble	from 1 to 10	slightly soluble	from 100 to 1000
soluble	from 10 to 30	very slightly soluble	from 1000 to 10,000

The term `partly soluble' is used to describe a mixture of which only some of the components dissolve and insoluble or practically insoluble means volume of solvent should be more than 10,000 ml/gm

If needed, slight acidification or alkalinization can be used to enhance solubility of weakly basic or acidic drug respectively. Similarly either warming (if it is not thermo labile) e.g. chloralose or cooling e.g. streptozotocin, can also be employed to solublise the drug.

2. Use of solvent- Double distilled water should be the first choice if solubility of dug allows it. However the solvent should be selected considering its effect on the living system, the cost of solvent, stability of solvent, solvent-solute interactions, applicability for parenteral administration etc. Many such solvents are used like- Saline, methanol, ethanol, propylene glycol, polyethylene glycol, DMF, DMSO etc. In case if it is to be administered by oral or intra-gastric route the drug can be suspended with suspending agent like acacia gum, sodium carboxy methyl cellulose (CMC) etc.

3. Cost of drug or availability of drug- If drug costly, little available (e.g. extracts) or necessitates use of costly solvent, the method is directed to use minimum possible weighable quantity to make solution. The dilutions to be made carefully.

4. Duration of use of drug- Whether it will be needed for short time (one-two days) or for longer time (for several days)

5. Stability of drug in solution- Several factors affect the stability of drug in solution of which   pH, temperature, light, presence metal ions (for oxidizing drugs) are the major factors. If above three factors allows drug to be freshly prepared, it automatically minimizes the difficulty. However, in circumstances where either solutions are to be preserved for long time or even in short duration the agents are liable for degradation, methods to minimizes the role of above mentioned factors can be applied like- maintaining pH e.g. Acetylcholine solution, keeping in refrigerator can protect all most all drug solutions and even solids form from ill effects of temperature and also by minimizing the actions other factors, chelators are added to prevent metal catalyzed oxidations. Many times antioxidants are added, if they are not affecting the response by direct or indirect action, to prevent auto oxidation of agents like catecholamines.

Pharmacologists must be acquainted with various facts related to various terms involved in measurement of various factors, their smaller and larger forms with conversions formulae, various forms of solutions and methods to make dilutions to obtain solution of appropriate concentration.

Various units and their variables are enlisted in **Table 2**. It is apt to note that they need to know the range from at least kilo to femto which are routinely encountered during routine laboratory work.

Mass versus volume

Mass can be determined at a precision of < 0.2 mg on a routine basis with an analytical balance and more precise instruments exist. Both solids and liquids are easily quantified by weighing.

The volume of a liquid is usually determined by calibrated glassware such as burettes and volumetric flasks. For very small volumes precision syringes are available. The use of graduated beakers and cylinders is not recommended as their indication of volume is not so accurate. The volume of solids, particularly of powders, is often difficult to measure, which is why mass is the more usual measure.

Concentration

There are a number of ways in which solution concentrations may be expressed. As a student who study science, the ability to defined concentration on molarity, molality, normality, mole fraction, and percentage as a part of the concentrations unit are must be have, because concentration units always be used in every science calculation, from this we can calculate masses and vice versa.

Table 2 Various Units of measurement with their prefixes denoting changes in the value

Prefix	Kilo	centi	deci	-	Milli	Micro	Nano	Pico	Femto	Atto	Zepto	Yocto
Times of given unit	10^3 x	10^2 x	10 x	1	10^{-3} x	10^{-6} x	10^{-9} x	10^{-12} x	10^{-15} x	10^{-18} x	10^{-21} x	10^{-24} x
Common Abbreviation	K	C	d		m	μ	N	P	F	A	Z	y
SI Units — Volume	L	μl	nl		ml	μl	nl	pl	Fl	al	zl	yl
SI Units — Mass	Kg	cg	dg	Gram (g)	mg	μg	ng	pg	Fg	ag	zg	yg
SI Units — Length	Mtr	μm	nm	Metre	mm	μm	nm	pm	Fm	am	zm	ym
SI Units — Time		60m=1Hr	60s=1min	Second	ms	μs	ns	ps	Fs	as	zs	ys
Solutions — Molar	Usually not needed			Molar	mM / 10^{-3} molar	μM / 10^{-6} molar	nM / 10^{-9} molar	pM / 10^{-12} molar	fM / 10^{-15} molar	aM / 10^{-18} molar	zM / 10^{-21} molar	yM / 10^{-24} molar

Molarity is the unit used to describe the number of moles of a chemical or compounds in one litre (L) of solution and is thus a unit of *concentration*. By this definition, a 1.0 Molar (1.0 M) solution is equivalent to one *formula weight* (FW = g/mole) or Molecular Weight of a compound dissolved it contains one mole of substance in each litre of the solution, it is prepared by dissolving one mole of substance in the solvent and diluting to a final volume of one litre in volumetric flask. Molarity has the unit of Molar that abbreviated as M.

Molality (m) is defined the number of moles in one kilogram of solvent. Remember we use mass of the solvent not the solution. A one molal solution contains one mole per 100 grams of solvent. Molal concentrations are not temperature dependent as molar and normal concentration since the solvent volume is temperature dependent.

Normality: A normal is one gram equivalent of a solute per litre of solution. The definition of a gram equivalent varies depending on the type of chemical reaction that is discussed - it can refer to acids, bases, redox species, and ions that will precipitate.

Mole fraction: The *mole fraction* X, (also called *molar fraction*) denotes the number of moles of solute as a proportion of the total number of moles in a solution. For instance: 1 mole of solute dissolved in 9 moles of solvent has a mole fraction of 1/10 or 0.1. Mole fractions are *dimensionless* quantities. (The *mole percentage* or *molar percentage*, denoted "mol %" and equal to 100% times the mole fraction, is sometimes quoted instead of the mole fraction.)

As both mole fractions and molality are only based on the masses of the components it is easy to convert between these measures. This is not true for molarity, which requires knowledge of the density.

Mass percentage (fraction): *Mass percentage* denotes the mass of a substance in a mixture as a percentage of the mass of the entire mixture. (Mass fraction x_m can be used instead of mass percentage by dividing mass percentage to 100.) For instance: if a bottle contains 35 grams of glycerin and 65 grams of water, then it contains 35% glycerin by mass or 0.35 mass fraction glycerin.

Mass-volume percentage: Mass-volume percentage, (sometimes referred to as weight-volume percentage or percent weight per volume and often abbreviated as % m/v or % w/v) describes the mass of the solute in g per 100 mL of the resulting solution. Mass-volume percentage is often used for solutions made from a solid solute dissolved in a liquid. For example, a 40% w/v sugar solution contains 40 g of sugar per 100 mL of resulting solution.

Volume-volume percentage: Volume-volume percentage (sometimes referred to as percent volume per volume and abbreviated as % v/v) describes the volume of the solute in mL per 100 mL of the resulting solution. This is most useful when a liquid - liquid solution is being prepared, although it is used for mixtures of gases as well. For example, a 40% v/v ethanol solution contains 40 mL ethanol per 100 mL total volume.

"Parts-per" Terms

The "Parts-per" term describes the amount of one substance in another and is thus related to the mass fraction. It is the ratio of the amount of the substance of interest to the amount of that substance plus the amount of the substance it is in.. It is used in some areas of science and engineering because it does not require conversion from weights or volumes to more chemically relevant units such as normality or molarity.

1. *Parts per hundred* (denoted by '%' [the per cent symbol], and very rarely 'pph') - denotes the amount of a given substance in a total amount of 100 regardless of the units of measure as long as they are the same. e.g. 1 gram per 100 gram. 1 part in 10^2.

2. *Parts per thousand* (denoted by '‰' [the per mille symbol], and occasionally 'ppt', but this usage can be confusing because it more often denotes parts per trillion) denotes the amount of a given substance in a total amount of 1000 regardless of the units of measure as long as they are the same. e.g. 1 milligram per gram, or 1 gram per kilogram. 1 part in 10^3.

3. *Parts per million* ('ppm') denotes the amount of a given substance in a total amount of 1,000,000 regardless of the units of measure used as long as they are the same. e.g. 1 milligram per kilogram. 1 part in 10^6.

4. *Parts per billion* ('ppb') denotes the amount of a given substance in a total amount of 1,000,000,000 regardless of the units of measure as long as they are the same. e.g. 1 milligram per tonne. 1 part in 10^9.

5. *Parts per trillion* ('ppt') denotes the amount of a given substance in a total amount of 1,000,000,000,000 regardless of the units of measure as long as they are the same. e.g. 1 milligram per kilotonne. 1 part in 10^{12}.

6. *Parts per quadrillion* ('ppq') denotes the amount of a given substance in a total amount of 1,000,000,000,000,000 regardless of the units of measure as long as they are the same. e.g. 1 milligram per megatonne. 1 part in 10^{15}.

How to Make Simple Solutions and Dilutions

It is also must for a Pharmacologist to know the various techniques to make various types of solutions and also how to make dilutions when ever required.

1. Simple Dilution (Dilution Factor Method based on ratios)

A *simple dilution* is one in which a *unit volume* of a liquid material of interest is combined with an appropriate volume of a *solvent* liquid to achieve the desired concentration. The *dilution factor* is the total number of unit volumes in which your material will be dissolved. e. g. 1: 6 dilution means adding 1 unit volume (part) of diluent (the material to be diluted) + 5 unit volumes (parts) of the solvent medium to yield 1/6 dilution of solution.

2. Serial Dilution

A *serial dilution* is simply a series of simple dilutions which leads to very dilute solution with very high dilution factor. The *total dilution factor* at any point is the *product* of the individual dilution factors in each step up to it as shown below-

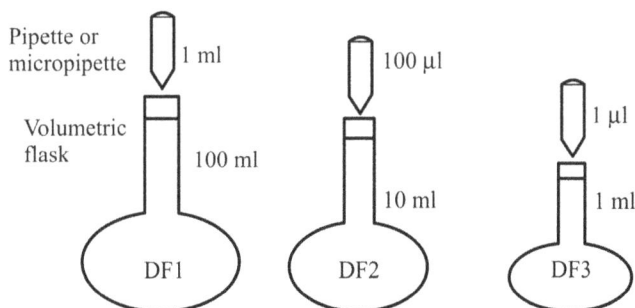

DF1=1 ml diluted to 100 ml= 100 times, DF2= 100 µl diluted to 10 ml= 100 times, DF3= 1 µl diluted 1 ml= 1000 times.

Final dilution factor (DF) = DF1 x DF2 x DF3 x .....x DFn (n-number of time dilutions are made)

This is most important method for obtaining solutions of drugs other chemicals with very small concentration like nanomolar (nM). This is particularly highly essential part in bioassays where solutions of various test and standard drugs to be prepared with different concentrations.

3. Calculations for modifications in concentrations

The equation given below helps in simple dilution to make desired volume of solution with desired concentration.

(stock solution attributes) $V_1C_1=V_2C_2$ (new solution attributes)

Example: Suppose you have 2 ml of a stock solution of 100 mg/ml Acetyl Choline (= C_1) and you want to make 500 µl (= V_2) of solution having 2.5 mg/ ml (= C_2). You need to know what volume (V_1) of the stock to use as part of the 500 µl total volume needed.

V_1 = the volume of stock solution required to be added to achieve desired concentration. **Unknown.**

C_1 = the stock solution available i.e. 100 mg/ ml in

V_2 = total volume needed at the new concentration = 500 µl = 0.5 ml

C_2 = the new concentration = 2.5 mg/ ml

By algebraic rearrangement:

$V_1 = (V_2 \text{ x } C_2) / C_1$

$V_1 = (0.5 \text{ ml x } 2.5 \text{ mg/ml}) / 100 \text{ mg/ml}$

$V_1 = 0.0125 \text{ ml, or } 12.50 \text{ ul}$

Thus 0.0125 ml i.e. 12.5 µl **of** 2.5 mg/ ml **stock solution** to be diluted with solvent sufficient to make the 500 µl of solution.

4. Moles and Molar solutions (unit = M = moles/L)

It is more convenient to use **molarity** when calculating concentrations. It helps to have drug solutions with molar concentrations during experiments conducted for calculating pA_2, pD_2 values.

To determine how many grams of reagent to use- Multiply the formula weight (FW) or Molecular Weight (MW) by the desired molarity (Z): **FW x Z moles/L = amount of solute**

To prepare a specific volume of a specific molar solution from a dry reagent

A chemical has a FW / MW of 167 g/mole and you need 50 ml (0.05 L) of 0.25 M solution. How many grams of the chemical must be dissolved in 40 ml (0.04 L) solvent to make this solution?

X grams/desired volume (L) = desired molarity (mole/L) x FW (g/mole) by algrebraic rearrangement,

X grams = desired volume (L) x desired molarity (mole/L) x FW (g/mole)

X grams = 0.04 L x 0.25 mole/L x 167 g/mole = 1.67 g

5. Percent Solutions (% = parts per hundred or grams/100 ml)

Many reagents are mixed as *percent concentrations* as weight per volume for dry reagent OR volume per volume for solutions. When working with a dry reagent it is mixed as *dry mass (g) per volume* and can be simply calculated as the *% concentration x volume needed = mass of reagent to use.*

To make 400 ml of saline i.e. (0.9 % NaCl =0.9/100=0.009) dissolve 0.009 x 400 = 3.6 g NaCl in 400 ml water.

When using **liquid reagents** the percent concentration is based upon *volume per volume (v/v)*, and is similarly calculated as *% concentration x volume needed = volume of reagent to use.*

To convert from % solution to molarity, multiply the % solution by 10 to express the percent solution grams/L, then divide by the formula weight.

$$\text{Molarity} = \frac{(\text{grams reagent} / 100 \text{ ml}) \times 10}{\text{FW}}$$

6. Concentrated stock solutions - using "X" units

Stock solutions of stable compounds are routinely maintained in labs as more concentrated solutions that can be diluted to working strength when used in typical applications. The usual working concentration is denoted as 1X. A solution 20 times more concentrated would be denoted as 20X and would require a 1:20 dilution to restore the typical working concentration.

3

Common Agonists and Antagonists

Most of the basics related to agonist, antagonist was discussed in previous chapter. It was clear that agonists act on receptors to elicit the response and antagonist prevent to do so. It is worthwhile to see some important receptor types as most cell-surface receptors fall into structurally-related types called super families. The members of super families exhibit structural similarities with minor variations reflecting in to diverse changes in the out come (response) through the receptor. Many such super families of receptors are identified with the help of biotechnology and other advanced sciences out of that most important are G-protein-linked receptors. It share a 7-helical structure that link to a second messenger through a G-protein and ligand-gated ion channels, in which the binding of the ligand directly changes an ionic conductance. In addition, some growth-factor receptors are linked to a tyrosine kinase enzyme. Other superfamilies have also been recognised e.g. nuclear receptors for steroids.

G-protein Coupled Receptors (GPCR)

The name is short for guanine nucleotide binding protein. These receptors are also called as metabotropic receptors. G proteins bind to the cytoplasmic face of the receptors which are a class of membrane proteins that causes the activation of a 7-helical receptor to the subsequent activation of its second messenger. They have three different subunits (α-, β- and γ - subunits which are tightly bound to each other hence called as heterotrimeric proteins. The α subunit is the GTP-binding subunit which confers specific recognition by receptor and effector. The direct signalling such as activation of inward rectifier K^+ (GIRK) channels and binding sites for G protein receptor kinases (GRKs). Activation of the G_a subunit by GTP allows it to both regulate an effector protein and drive the release of G_{bg} subunits, which not only regulate their own group of effectors but also reassociate with GDP-liganded G_a to return the system back to the initial normal state.

Large variety of GPCRs are known out of which many can be grouped into categories depending on which second messenger they predominantly control. Thus, G_s frequently activates adenylyl cyclase to produce cyclic Adenine Mono Phosphate a Second messenger, whereas G_i inhibits it; G_q

mediates the stimulation of phospholipase C and hence phosphoinositide turnover to form Inositol Tri Phosphate (IP_3) and Di Acyl Glycerol (DAG). However, these may not always true- many G proteins do not necessarily couple to the same second messenger in different cells, and they may even couple to more than one in a single cell.

Gs protein is irreversibly activated by cholera toxin. Subtypes of Gi protein have been identified, some of which are irreversibly inactivated by pertussis toxin by ADP-ribosylation of the α-subunit in both instances.

The 7-transmembrane domain receptor- Schematic diagram of a 7-transmembrane domain receptor depicting ligand binding sites and cellular mechanism sites.

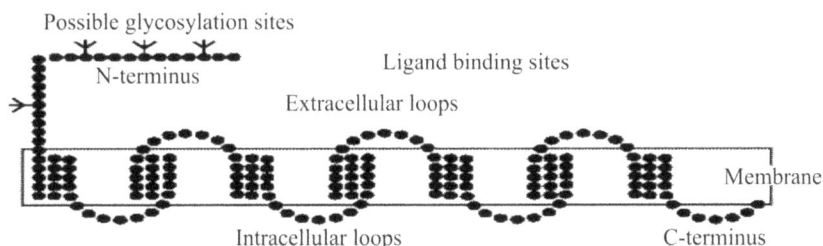

Cellular mechanism sites-second messanger, ion channel etc.

The filled circles represent amino acid residues which make a sequence spanning 7 units linked by 3 extracellular and 3 intracellular loops. The third intracellular loop links to the G-protein; often the ligand binding site is found within the space enclosed by the transmembrane loops and/or extracellular domains as shown in figure. The following receptors have been identified to have 7TM structure: Acetyl Choloine-(muscarinic) M_1, M_2, M_3, M_4 and M_5 receptors, Adreno CorticoTropic Hormone-ACTH, Adenosine- A_1, A_{2a}, A_{2b} and A_3, α_{1A}-, α_{1B}-, α_{1C}-, α_{2A}-, α_{2B}-, α_{2C}-, α_{2D}-, β_1-, β_2- and β_3-adrenoceptors, Angiotensin- AT_{1A} and AT_{1B}, arg-vasopressin, bombesin/gastrin releasing peptide, bradykinin B2, calcitonin, cannabinoid receptor, CCKA, CCKB, complement anaphylotoxin C5a, Dopamine- D_1 (A and B), D_2, D_3, D_4 and D_5 receptors, Endothelin- ET_A and ET_B, FSH, GAB_{AB}, 6- glutamate metabotropic receptors, GonadoTropic Releasing Hormone-GnRH, Histamine- H_1 and H_2, interleukin IL-8, LH, neurokinin NK1, NK2 and NK3, neurotensin, Neuropeptide Y-NPY, opioid, oxytocin, prostaglandin EP_3, secretin, Serotonin (5- Hydroxy Tryptamine) $5HT_{1A}$, $5HT_{1B}$, $5HT_{1D}$ (α and β), $5HT_{1E}$, $5HT_2$, $5HT_{2C}$ and $5HT_4$ receptors, somatostatin TR_1, TR_2 and TR_3, thrombin, thromboxane, TRH and TSH.

Enzyme-linked receptors

(a) Tyrosine kinase linked- These include the intrinsic type of receptors which constitutes insulin receptor and growth factor receptors such as epidermal growth factor (EGF) and platelet-derived growth factor (PDGF).

(b) Extrinsic Receptors- These are receptor playing role in signal transduction like MAPK, JAK, STAT etc.

Ion-channel-linked receptors

This class of receptor are linked to ion-channels, the conductance of which is modulated by the binding of agonists or antagonists. This superfamily includes the nicotinic acetylcholine receptor, the GABAA and glycine receptors, the 5HT3 receptor, the purine P2X receptor and some excitatory amino-acid receptors. The receptors consist of subunits, each having four transmembrane domains, which form complexes of varying stoichiometry. Many variant forms of subunit have been discovered, although the implications of this for defining receptor subtypes are not yet clear.

Ion-channels

There are four identified types of ion-channel through which calcium, potassium, sodium or chloride ions selectively cross the membrane. Some information on calcium and potassium channels, responsible for effect of some drugs, is outlined below.

Calcium channels

(a) Voltage-dependent calcium channels

L-type – They have large unit conductance (25pS) and activated by high membrane potentials. They are slowly inactivated by Ca^{2+}-dependent/ voltage-dependent mechanisms. These types of channels are predominantly present in muscle cells and mediate contraction in cardiac and smooth muscle cells. These are activated by Bay K-8644, CGP 28392 and verapamil, dihydropyridines (e.g. Nifedipine; Amlodepine etc) and diltiazem causes blocking (Popularly called as Calcium Channel Blockers)

N-type – They have intermediate unit conductance (12-20pS) and activated by high membrane potentials. The membrane potentials more positive than -40mV leads to inactivation of channel. They are mainly located on neurons to control neurotransmitter release and blocked by ω-conotoxin.

P-type - They have intermediate unit conductance (10-12pS) and activated at moderately high membrane potentials. They are very slowly inactivated once membrane potentials become more positive than −40 mV. They are mainly neuronal and control neurotransmitter release (with N-type) but blocked by funnel web spider toxin ω-aga-IVA.

T-type - They have small unit conductance (8pS) and activated at relatively negative membrane potentials. They allow Transient Ca^{2+} current. Determine frequency of action potential generation in neurones and cardiac muscle cells. Antiepileptic agents like Ethosuximide, gabapentin, valproic acid block this channel.

(b) Receptor-operated calcium channels

Receptor activation, rather than membrane potential, is the main trigger for opening these channels.

(c) Intracellularly-activated Ca^{2+}-selective channels

Ryanodyne receptors- Ca^{2+} release channels in the sarcoplasmic reticulum, which release calcium for smooth muscle contraction Inositol-1, 4, 5-triphosphate (IP_3) receptors- Activated by elevated intracellular levels of IP_3 following stimulation of cell surface receptors. They are structurally similar to ryanodine receptors and also cause a release of intracellular calcium stores.

Potassium channels

(a) Voltage-dependent potassium channels

Derived from a large gene family whose diversity of channel properties may arise from alternative splicing or post-translational modifications. These channels are associated with a number of well characterised currents: delayed rectifier, transient outward and inward rectifier.

(b) Calcium-activated potassium channels

Three currents have been associated with this type of potassium channel: the large, the intermediate and the small conductance currents.

(c) ATP-sensitive potassium channels

ATP has been found to inhibit the opening of some potassium channels through which the IK (ATP) current flows. Such channels are inward-rectifying and voltage dependent.

(d) Receptor-linked potassium channels

Some potassium channels are opened by muscarinic receptor activation through coupling to a G-protein. The M-current is associated with such channels.

Sodium Channels

Voltage Gated Sodium Channels- Many class of drugs are known to act on it e.g. local anaesthetics, anti arrhythmic agents (Class-I) and some anti epileptics.

Intra Cellular Receptors

The receptors discussed before this section were acting on membrane receptors. In this type of receptors the ligand must enter the cell in active form and bind these intra cellular receptors.

These receptors are located inside the cell and most of the times present in nucleus (hence referred as nuclear receptors) while some times they may present on organelles. The Nuclear receptors cause modulation of gene expression (increase or decrease in replication, transcription like nuclear activities). e. g. Receptors for steroids. The activities regulated through these receptors are usually slow and long lasting as compared to membranous receptors.

Section-II

In this section brief information about some Neurotransmitters and/or other chemical signalling agents is to enable reader to have basic information before going for next sections which describe effect of one or other while explaining the topic. The information is brief and it advised to readers to have thorough reading of Pharmacology Books before going for experimental pharmacology.

1. **ACETYLCHOLINE (ACh):** One of the most important neurotransmitters and signalling agent, major constituent of Autonomous Nervous System (ANS) acting on autonomic ganglia and parasympathetic branch of ANS. It is also observed in CNS and plays important role in Parkinson and Alzheimer's disease. This is the transmitter responsible for skeletal muscle contraction.

Category	Chemicals/ Enzymes	Agents affecting activity
Precursors:	Choline and acetyl-CoA	Hemicholinium inhibit uptake of Choline
Synthesising enzymes:	Choline acetyl transferase	Vesamicol inhibit vesicular uptake
Metabolising enzymes:	Acetylcholinesterase (AChE)	Many AChE Inhibitors- Increases ACh actions-Reversible-
Metabolite:	Choline and acetate	Physostigmine, Neostigmine (Eserine) and OraganoPhosphorus compounds (irreversible). AChE reactivators- Pralidoxime etc to treat poisoning with AChEIs.

Botulinus and tetanus toxin inhibit the release while black widow spider toxin causes depletion to excessive release.

	M_1 ('neural')	M_2 ('cardiac')	M_3 ('glandular/ smooth muscle')	M_4	M_5
Type	GPCR (Metabotropic) Gq-	GPCR (Metabotropic) Gi	GPCR (Metabotropic) Gq-	GPCR (Metabotropic) Gi	GPCR (Metabotro pic) Gq
Effector Pathway	Excitatory- ↑IP₃, DAG- Depolarisation, ↓K+ conductance	Inhibitory- ↓cAMP ↓Ca²⁺ & ↓K⁺ conductance	Excitatory- ↑IP₃, Stimulation, ↑[Ca²⁺]ᵢ	Inhibitory- ↓cAMP	Excitatory ↑IP₃
Main locations	Cerebral cortex, Autonomic ganglia Glands: gastric, salivary, etc.	Heart: atria CNS: widely distributed	CNS, Blood vessels: endothelium Exocrine glands: gastric, salivary, etc. Smooth muscle: eye, airways, bladder, gastrointestinal tract.	CNS	CNS: substantia nigra, Salivary glands Iris/ciliary muscle
Effect	CNS excitation (slow epsp), memory () Gastric secretion	Inhibitory: Cardiac, Neural Central muscarinic effects (e.g. tremor, hypothermia)	Gastric, salivary secretion Gastrointestinal smooth muscle contraction, Ocular accommodation Vasodilatation	Enhanced locomotion	NA
Agonists (Non Selective)	Acetylcholine, Carbachol Oxotremorine	Acetylcholine Methacholine , Carbachol Oxotremorine			
Agonists (Selective)	*McNA343, Talsaclidine*				
Antagonists (non-selective)	Atropine , Dicycloverine, Tolterodine, Oxybutynin, Ipratropium				
Antagonists (selective	Pirenzepine, Maa toxin MT7 telenzepine	Hiacine, methoctramine	Darifenacin Hexahydrosiladif enidol	Ipratropium Maa toxin MT3, Tropicamide	

	Muscle type	Ganglion type		CNS type
Type	Ion Channel (Pentamer)	Ion Channel (Pentamer)	Ion Channel (Pentamer)	Ion Channel (Pentamer)
Effector Pathway	Excitatory-↑ cation permeability (mainly Na^+, K^+)	Excitatory-↑ cation permeability (mainly Na^+, K^+)	Pre- and postsynaptic excitation, ↑ cation permeability (mainly Na^+, K^+)	Pre- and postsynaptic excitation, ↑d Ca^{2+} permeability
location	neuromuscular junction: mainly postsynaptic	Autonomic ganglia: mainly postsynaptic	Many brain regions: pre- and postsynaptic	Many brain regions: pre- and postsynaptic
Agonists	Acetylcholine Carbachol Succinylcholine	Dimethylphenyl piperazinium Acetylcholine, Carbachol, Nicotine,	Acetylcholine, Nicotine Epibatidine, Cytosine	Dimethylphenylpi perazinium, Epibatidine,
Antagonists	Tubocurarine Pancuronium Atracurium Vecuronium α-Bungarotoxin α-Conotoxin	Mecamylamine Trimethaphan Hexamethonium α-Conotoxin	Mecamylamine Methylaconitine	α-Bungarotoxin α-Conotoxin Methylaconitine

2. **Norepinephrine (Noradrenaline; NE) and Epinephrine (Adrenaline; E) - Most** important neurotransmitters and signaling agents, hormones from adrenal medulla, neurotransmitter of sympathetic branch of ANS released at effector organs. It is also observed in CNS and plays important role in Depression and Psychoses.

Category	Chemicals/ Enzymes	Agents affecting activity
Precursors:	L-Tyrosine (a) -> L-DOPA (b) -> dopamine, (c) -> noradrenaline (d) -> adrenaline	α-Methyl DOPA – gets incorporated instead of normal constituent and produces false transmitter, show sypatholytic action
Synthesising enzymes:	(a) tyrosine hydroxylase, (b) L-aromatic amino-acid decarboxylase, (c) dopamine-beta-hydroxylase, (d) phenyl lethanolamine-N-methyl transferase	α-methyltyrosine- causes depletion of NA due to inhibition of enzymes.
Metabolising enzymes:	MAO and COMT	MAO inhibitors-Selegelene, Pargylene, Moclebamide and COMT inhibitors Tolcapone, entacapone are clinically used.
Metabolites:	Vanillylmandelic acid (VMA) and 3-methoxy-4-hydroxyphenylglycol (MHPG)	The levels of these metabolites are measured for diagnosis of adrenal tumors and excessive sympathetic activity

In addition there are several peculiarities in adrenergic transmission.

1. The synthesized NE/AD vesicularised using vesicular pump. This provides packed vesicle ready for exocytosis at the time of release and prevent degradation by MAO in the neuron. Reserpine blocks the pump and prevents vesiculariztion depleting neurotransmitter in vesicle and allowing degradation by MAO. Simultaneous administration of MAO inhibitor results in Reserpine reversal.

2. There are 2 major uptakes which removes catecholamines from the synapse uptake 1- the presynaptic neuron takes back the released catecholamine and Guanethidine etc block it while uptake-2 is infiltration of catecholamine in either surrounding tissues e.g. glial cells in CNS or postsynaptic neuron and Tricyclic antidepressants are believed to act through the mechanism.

Details-	α_1	α_2	β_1	β_2	β_3
Type	GPCR	GPCR	GPCR	GPCR	GPCR
Effector Pathway	PLC activation, $\uparrow$IP$_3$ $\uparrow$DAG, $\uparrow$Ca^{2+}	$\downarrow$cAMP, $\downarrow$Calcium channels, $\uparrow$Potassium channels	$\uparrow$cAMP	$\uparrow$cAMP	$\uparrow$cAMP
Heart Rate	Not Aware (NA)	NA	$\uparrow$	$\uparrow$	NA
Force of contraction	NA	NA	$\uparrow$	$\uparrow$	NA
Blood vessels	Constrict	Constrict/dilate	NA	Dilate	NA
Bronchi	Constrict	NA	NA	Dilate	NA
Gastrointestinal tract	Relax	Relax (presynaptic effect)	NA	Relax	NA
Gastrointestinal sphincters	Contract	NA	NA	NA	NA
Uterus	Contract	NA	NA	Relax	NA
Bladder detrusor	NA	NA	NA	Relax	NA
Bladder sphincter	Contract	NA	NA	NA	NA
Seminal tract	Contract	NA	NA	Relax	NA
Iris (radial muscle)	Contract	NA	NA	NA	NA
Ciliary muscle	NA	NA	NA	Relax	NA
Liver	Glycogenolysis	NA	NA	Glycogenolysis	NA
Fat	NA	NA	NA	NA	Lipolysis & Thermogenesis

Contd....

Skeletal muscle	NA	NA	NA	Tremor, muscle mass and speed of contraction ↑, Glycogenolysis	Thermogenesis
Selective agonists	Noradrenaline (NA) and Adrenaline		Isoprenaline		
Selective agonists (Sub Class)	Phenylephrine, methoxamine	Clonidine, clenbuterol	Dobutamine, xamoterol	Salbutamol, terbutaline salmeterol, formoterol	BRL 37344
Selective antagonists	Prazosin, doxazocin	Yohimbine, idazoxan	Atenolol , metoprolol	Butoxamine	
Predominance	NE ≥E >>ISO	E >NE >>ISO	ISO >NE >E	ISO > E > NE	ISO >NE = E

3. **DOPAMINE (DA) - Dopamine** is earlier believed to be just precursor of epinephrine but it is know confirmed to have own identity as neurotransmitter at central and peripheral nervous system. Central effects are prominent and many drugs acting on Dopaminergic system are therapeutically available.

Category	Chemicals/ Enzymes	Agents affecting activity
Precursors:	Tyrosine (a) -> L- dihydroxyphenyl alanine (L-DOPA), (b) -7gt; dopamine	L- DOPA –Is used as precursor of Dopamine in Parkinson Disease.
Synthesising enzymes:	(a) Tyrosine hydroxylase; (b) L-aromatic aminoacid decarboxylase (DOPA decarboxylase)	Pyridoxin can cause ↑ in Dopa decarboxylase activity. Carbidopa blocks peripheral Dopa Decarboxylase.
Metabolising enzymes:	MAO and catechol-O-methyl transferase (COMT)	MAO inhibitors-Selegelene, Pargylene, Moclebamide and COMT inhibitors Tolcapone, entacapone are clinically used.
Metabolites:	3,4-Dihydroxyphenylacetic acid (DOPAC) and homovanillic acid (HVA)	

Detail's	D_1 Family		D_2 Family		
	D_1	D_5	D_2	D_3	D_4
Type	GPCR Gs	GPCR Gs	GPCR Gi	GPCR Gi	GPCR Gi
Effector Pathway	↑ cAMP,	↑ cAMP,	↓ cAMP (↑) $K+$ / ↓ Ca^{++}	?	?
Effect	Mainly postsynaptic Inhibitory	Pre and postsynaptic inhibition, regulation of hormone release	Autoreceptors, Vomiting, Psychosis.		Neuronal circuits
Agonists	SKF 38393	Dopamine	Quinpirole	7-OH-DPAT	Dopamine
Antagonists	Sch 23390	Sch 23390	Sulpiride	AJ-76	Clozapine

4. **PROSTANOIDS   (Prostaglandins,   prostacyclin-   PG   and thromboxane-TX) and Leucotrienes (LT)** – Known as mediators of inflammation and products of Arachidonic acid metabolism. Several products are formed which play important role in many physiological and pathological conditions. Only few are discussed here.

Category	Chemicals/ Enzymes for PG	Chemicals/ Enzymes for LT	Agents affecting activity for PG	Agents affecting activity for LT
Precursors:	Arachidonic acid (i.e. eicosatetraenoic acid; 2-series prostanoids), eicosatrinoic and eicosapentaenoic acids		Glucocorticoids inhibiting PL-A$_2$.	
Synthesising enzymes:	Prostaglandin synthetase (cyclooxygen-ase -COX), PGI$_2$ synthase, TX synthase.	5-Lipoxygenase (LPO)	COX inhibitors like selective-Rofecoxib etc, Non-Selective-Ibuprofen, Diclofenac etc and Aspirin (TX inhibition)	Zileuton is 5-LPO
Metabolising enzymes:	15-hydroxyprostagla ndin dehydrogenase, PG-9-keto-reductase	LTB 12-hydroxydehydr ogenase	Significantly important information is not available.	
Metabolites:	large number of oxidized metabolites	12-oxo-LTB$_4$		

A. **Prostaglandin (PG):** These were believed as products of inflammatory cascade and however known for many physiological activities.

| Detail's | DP (PGD(2)) | EP (PGE(2)), subdivided as shown | | | FP (PGF(2-α)) | IP (PGI(2)) | TP (TXA(2)) |
		EP(1)	EP(2)	EP(3)			
Type	GPCR(G$_i$)	GPCR G$_q$	GPCR	GPCR	GPCR G$_q$	GPCR	GPCR
Effector Pathway	↑ cAMP, ↑ Ca^{2+} $_i$	IP3	↑cAMP	IP3, cAMP	IP3	↑cAMP	PLC-IP$_3$–Ca^{2+}
Location	platelets, vasculature, lung, smooth muscles	platelets, vasculature, lung, smooth muscles	platelets, vasculature, lung, smooth muscles	GI tract	kidney, heart, lung, stomach, and eye; it is most abundant in the corpus luteum	many tissues and cells, including human kidney, lung, spine, liver, vasculature, and heart.	platelets, vasculature, lung, kidney, heart, thymus, and spleen
Effects	Vasodilation, ↓platelet aggregatrion, Relax brochial, GI smooth muscle	Constrict brochial, GI smooth muscle	Vasodilation, Relax brochial, GI smooth muscle. ↑ secretion	↑ mucus secretion,	Myometrial contractions	Vasodilation	Platelet aggregation
Agonists	BW245C, ZK110841	sulprostone, iloprost	AY23626, butaprost, rioprostil	Sulproston e, enprostil, rioprostil, AY23626, GR 63799	fluprostenol, cloprostenol	iloprost, cicaprost	U-46619, STA2, EP171
Antagonists	BWA868C, AH6809	AH6809, SC-19220	none	none	none	none	GR32191, SQ28668 BM13505, EP092,

B. Leucotrienes

Details	BLT		cysteinyl-containing
	BLT_1	BLT_2	leucotrienes Cyst LT
Type	GPCR G_{16}, G_i	GPCR G_q-like, G_i-like, G_z-like	GPCR
Effector Pathway			IP_3
Location	leukocytes, spleen, neutrophils		Resp System, CVS
Effects	inflammatory response, Chemotaxis, ↑ proliferation; cytokine release; free radical release		Spasmogenic, ↓ BP
Agonists	LTB_4		LTC_4 LTD_4, LTE_4, LTF_4 *sulfidopeptide*
Antagonists	NA		Zafirlukast, Montelukast

4. **HISTAMINE (HA):** Histamine was earlier identified as important mediator of inflammation. However gastric and other activities are indicative of its other roles as signalling molecule.

Category	Chemicals/ Enzymes	Agents affecting activity
Precursors:	Histidine	Significantly important information is not available.
Synthesising enzymes:	Histidine decarboxylase	
Metabolising enzymes:	Histamine-N-methyl transferase, histaminase, histamine acetylase, diamine oxidase	
Metabolite:	Methylhistamine, imidazolyl acetic acid, N-methyl imidazolyl acetic acid	

Details	H_1	H_2	H_3
Type	GPCR G_q/G_{11}	GPCR G_s,	GPCR
Effector Pathway	elevates IP3 turnover	elevates cAMP	(? ↓ coupling to PLC; ?Ca^{2+})
Location	Blood vessels, Smooth muscles	Gastric glands	terminals as well as on cell bodies/dendrites in the hypothalamic tuberomammillary nucleus on histaminergic neurons
Effects	Vasodilation. constriction	Acid Secretion	depresses neuronal firing
Agonists	2-(3-fluorophenyl) histamine, 2-[(3-trifluoromethyl) phenyl] histamine	amthamine, impromidine	(R)-α-methylhistamine, imetit (S-[2-4(5)-imidazolyl]ethylis othiourea)
Antagonists	Mepyramine, triprolidine	ranitidine tiotidine	clobenpropit, thioperamide

5. NITRIC OXIDE (NO; formerly EDRF- Endothelium Derived Relaxing Factor)

Category	Chemicals/ Enzymes	Agents affecting activity
Precursors:	L-arginine	Significantly important information is not available.
Synthesising enzymes:	NO Synthase (NOS)- Constitutive- eNOS, nNOS and Inducible iNOS	L-NMMA and L-NAME, Aminoguanidine (iNOS inhibitor)
Metabolising enzymes:	none: diffusion and spontaneous breakdown	The Phospho diasterase enzyme (PDE-V) shortens the action by metabolising cGMP. Sildenafil increases action by inhibiting PDE.
Metabolite:	$NO_{(2)}^-$, $NO_{(3)}^-$	Nitrate levels are used for estimation

NO has no conventional receptor, but it activates guanylate cyclase directly. The transduction mechanism involves cGMP – Protein Kinase. NO can be generated by nitrates glyceryl trinitrate or sodium nitroprusside.

6. Serotonin

Category	Chemicals/ Enzymes	Agents affecting activity
Precursors:	L-Tryptophan -> 5-HydroxyTryptophan- 5-HT	Tryptophan increases the 5- HT level
Synthesising enzymes:	(a) Trypotophan hydroxylase, (b) L-aromatic amino-acid decarboxylase,	p-Clorophenyl alanine blocks 5-HT synthesis and very toxic
Metabolising enzymes:	MAO and COMT	Mao-A I –Tranycypromine and MAO-B IChorgyline
Metabolite:	5-Hydroxy indole acetic acid	Diagnosis of carcinoid syndrome.

Although structurally different it exhibits similarity with catecholamines in reuptakes and vesicular storage. Accordingly Tricyclic antidepressants and reserpine like drugs will also play role in serotonigeric transmission. The metabolising enzymes are also same.

Details	5-HT$_{1A}$	5-HT$_{1B}$	5-HT$_{1D}$	5-HT$_{2A}$	5-HT$_{2B}$	5-HT$_{2C}$
Type	GPCR	GPCR	GPCR	GPCR	GPCR	GPCR
Effector Pathway	↓cAMP, ↑ K$^+$, ↓Ca	↓cAMP	↓cAMP	↑IP$_3$/DAG	↑IP$_3$/DAG	↑IP$_3$/DAG
Location	CNS	CNS, Vascular smooth muscle	CNS, Blood vessels	Platelets, CNS, PNS, Smooth muscle	Gastric fundus	CNS Choroid plexus
Effects	Neuronal Inhibitory Behavioural effects: anxiety, sleep, feeding, thermoregulation.	Inhibitory Presynaptic, Behavioural effects Pulmonary vasoconstriction	Cerebral vasoconstriction Behavioural effects: locomotion	Behavioural effects, Neuronal excitation, Smooth muscle contraction (gut, bronchi, etc.), Platelet aggregation, Vasoconstriction/vas odilatation	Contraction	Cerebrospinal fluid secretion
Non Selective Agonists	5-CT			α-Me-5-HT LSD (CNS) LSD (periphery)		
Selective Agonists	8-OH-DPAT Buspirone (PA)	Ergotamine (PA)	Sumatriptan			
Antagonist	Methiothepin, Spiperone Ergotamine (PA)	Ergotamine (PA)	Ergotamine (PA)	Pizotifen (non-selective) Ketanserin, Cyproheptadine, Methysergide	-	Methysergide de

Details	5-HT$_3$	5-HT$_4$	5-HT$_5$	5-HT$_6$	5-HT$_7$
Type	ligand-gated cation channel	GPCR	GPCR	GPCR	GPCR
Effector Pathway	None	↑cAMP	NA	NA	↑cAMP
Location	CNS, PNS	CNS, PNS (GI tract)	CNS	CNS	CNS, GI tract, Blood vessels
Effects	Emesis, Behavioural effects: anxiety Neuronal excitation (autonomic, nociceptive neurons)	Neuronal excitation, GI motility	NA	NA	NA
Agonists	2-Me-5-HT, Chlorophenyl-biguanide	Tegaserod, 5-Methoxy-tryptamine, Metoclopramide	NA	NA	5-CT LSD No selective agonist
Antagonists	Ondansetron, Tropisetron, Granisetron	Various experimental compounds (e.g. GR113808, SB207266)	NA	NA	Various 5-HT$_2$ antagonists No selective antagonists

7. g-AMINOBUTYRIC ACID (GABA)-

Category	Chemicals/ Enzymes	Agents affecting activity
Precursors:	Glutamate	Significantly important information is not available.
Synthesising enzymes:	Glutamic acid decarboxylase (GAD)	
Metabolising enzymes:	GABA transaminase	Many antiepileptic drugs inhibit the enzyme e.g. Valproic acid,
Metabolite:	Succinic semialdehyde	

Details	GABA$_A$			GABA$_B$
	GABA$_A$ Receptor site	Benzodiazepine site (Modulatory)	Modulatory site (others)	
Type	Ligand Gated Ion Channel (↑) Cl			GPCR;
Effector mechanism	None			↑K+, (↓) Ca2+, (↓)cAMP
Location	Widespread in CNS many GABAergic interneurons playing role.			Pre- and postsynaptic Widespread
Effects	Postsynaptic Inhibitory (fast ipsp). Reduction in impulse conduction and neurotransmitter (NT) release.			Presynaptic Inhibitory (↓ Ca^{2+} entry) Postsynaptic inhibition (↑ K$^+$ permeability)
Endogenous agonist	GABA	?Diazepam-binding inhibitor	Various neurosteroids (e.g. progesterone metabolites)	GABA
Other agonist	Muscimol Gaboxadol (THIP, partial agonist) isoguvacin	Anxiolytic benzodiazepines (e.g. diazepam)	Barbiturates Steroid anaesthetics (e.g. αxolone)	Baclofen, CGP 97541
Antagonist	Bicuculline Gabazine	Flumazenil	NA	2-OH-Saclofen, Phaclofen, CGP 35348
Channel blocker	Picrotoxin	NA	NA	NA

8.   GLUTAMATE (and ASPARTATE)

Category	Chemicals/ Enzymes	Agents affecting activity
Precursors:	None	Significantly important information is not available.
Synthesising enzymes:	None	
Metabolising enzymes:	Glutamate transaminase (uptake is more important)	
Metabolite:	Glutamine	

Details	NMDA	AMPA	Kainate	Metabotropic
Type	Ligand-gated cation channel (slow kinetics, high Ca^{2+} permeability)	Ligand-gated cation channel (fast kinetics; show low Ca^{2+} permeability)	Ligand-gated cation channel (fast kinetics, low Ca^{2+} permeability)	GPCR
Effector mechanism	None	None	None	IP_3-DAG-Ca^{2+}
Location	Postsynaptic (also glial) Wide distribution	Postsynaptic	Pre- and postsynaptic	Pre- and postsynaptic
Effects	Slow epsp Synaptic plasticity (long-term potentiation, long-term depression) Excitotoxicity	Fast epsp Wide distribution	Fast epsp ? Presynaptic Inhibitory Limited distribution	Synaptic modulation Excitotoxicity
Endogenous agonist	Glutamate Aspartate	Glutamate	Glutamate	Glutamate
Other agonist	NMDA	AMPA Quisqualate	Kainate Domoate	D-AP4, ACPD, 1S,3R-ACPD, ibotenate
Antagonist	AP-5, AP-7, CGS 19755 (selfotel) CPP, LY 235959, CGP37849	NBQX, CNQX, LY 293558, DNQX	NBQX, LY 377770	MCPG
Other modulator	Polyamines (e.g. spermine, spermidine), Mg^{2+}, Zn^{2+}	Cyclothiazide Aniracetam Ampakines Piracetam	-	-
Channel blocker	Dizocilpine (MK801), Phencyclidine, Ketamine, Remacemide, Memantine, Mg^{2+}	-	-	Not applicable

9. GLYCINE

Category	Chemicals/ Enzymes
Precursors:	None
Synthesising enzymes:	None
Metabolising enzymes:	None (uptake is more important)
Metabolite:	None

	Glycine	Allosteric *Modulatory* site on NMDA receptor *(glycine)*
Type	Ligand-gated chloride channel	Ligand-gated cation channel (slow kinetics, high Ca^{2+} permeability)
Effector mechanism(s)	None	None
Location	Postsynaptic Mainly in brain stem and spinal cord	As modulatory site on NMDA receptor
Effects	Postsynaptic Inhibitory (fast ipsp)	The glycine binding is important for activation of NMDA receptor
Endogenous agonist	Glycine β-Alanine Taurine	Glycine, D-Serine
Other agonist	-	Cycloserine
Antagonist	Strychnine	7-Chloro-kynurenic acid, ACEA 1021, HA-466

10.   Purinergic Receptors- ADENOSINE (P1 purinoceptors), ATP (P$_2$ purinoceptors) and ADP

(a)   Adenosine

Category	Chemicals/ Enzymes	Agents affecting activity
Precursors:	Mainly AMP (from released ATP)	Significantly important information is not available.
Synthesising enzymes:	Mainly 5'-nucleotidase	
Metabolising enzymes:	Adenosine deaminase	
Metabolite:	Inosine	

Details	P$_1$ Family			
	A$_1$	A$_2$A	A$_2$B	A$_3$
Type	GPCR	GPCR	GPCR	GPCR
Effector Pathway	($\downarrow$)cAMP	($\uparrow$)cAMP	($\uparrow$)cAMP	($\downarrow$)cAMP
Location	Smooth muscles, Neurons	Tissues,	Blood vessels, tissues	Mast cell, bronchial smooth muscle
Effects	Bronchoconstriction, $\downarrow$ NT release	Nociception,	Adenosine release,	release of mediators Bronchoconstriction,
Agonists	CPA, R-PIA, GR 79236	CGS21680, CV-1808	Metrifudil	R-PIA, NECA
Antagonists	8PT, DPCPX	8PT, CGS 15943	8PT	none

B. Purinergic (ATP and ADP)

Category	Chemicals/ Enzymes	Agents affecting activity
Precursors:	Normal cellular constituent; formed from ADP	Significantly important information is not available.
Synthesising enzymes:	Phosphorylases	
Metabolising enzymes:	Phosphatases	
Metabolite:	ADP, AMP, adenosine, inosine	

Details	P_{2X}	P_{2Y}	P_{2T} (platelet)	P_{2Z} (mast cell)	P_{2U}
Type	GPCR	GPCR	GPCR	GPCR	GPCR
Effector Pathway	($\uparrow$) (cation) or (up) Ca^{2+}	IP3, ($\uparrow$) K	($\downarrow$) cAMP, ($\uparrow$)(cation)	?	IP3
Location	Smooth muscle, brain	Many tissues	NA	NA	NA
Effects	NA	NA	NA	NA	NA
Agonists	beta-gamma-Me-ATP	ADP-beta-F, 2-Me-S-ATP	ADP	ATP^{4-}	UTP
Antagonists	α-beta-Me-ATP (desensitises), suramin	Reactive blue 2, suramin	Suramin, AMP	none	none

11.   BRADYKININ (BK)

Category	Chemicals/ Enzymes	Agents affecting activity
Precursors:	Kininogens	Significantly important information is not available.
Synthesising enzymes:	Kallikrein	
Metabolising enzymes:	ACE, kininase I, (carboxypeptidase-N)	ACE I – induces coughing due to inhibition of ACE
Metabolite:	Des-Arg9-bradykinin, other fragments	

Details	B_1	B_2
Type	GPCR	GPCR
Effector Pathway	?	IP_3-DAG-Ca^{2+}
Location	Tissues, neurons	Tissues, neurons
Effects	Hyper algesia, cough	Pain Inflammation
Agonists	Des-Arg^9-BK	Hyp^9,Tyr(Me)^8-BK
Antagonists	Des-Arg^9, Leu^8-BK Des-Arg^{10}-HOE140	NPC567, HOE140, NPC349

12.   Endothelin

Category	Chemicals/ Enzymes	Agents affecting activity
Precursors:	preproET-1 etc.	Significantly important information
Synthesising enzymes:	"endothelin converting enzyme"	is not available.
Metabolising enzymes:	NA	
Metabolite:	NA	

Details	$ET_{(A)}$	$ET_{(B)}$	$ET_{(C)}$
Type	GPCR	GPCR	GPCR
Effector Pathway	IP_3-DAG-Ca^{2+}	IP_3-DAG-Ca^{2+}	?
Location	Smooth muscle,	Smooth muscle	
Function	Vaso and broncho constriction	Vasodilation, ↓ platelet aggregation	
Agonists	ET-1, ET-2	Sarafotoxin S6C, $[Ala^{(1),(3),(11),(15)}]$ ET-1, BQ 3020	
Antagonists	FR139317, BQ123, Bosentan	IRL 1038	

13.   Angiotensin

Category	Chemicals/ Enzymes	Agents affecting activity
Precursors:	Angiotensinogen, Angiotensin-I	
Synthesising enzymes:	Renin, Angiotensin Converting Enzyme (ACE)	Renin-Prostaglandins, β-receptor agonist, antagonist, ACE-I, captopril, enalapril. Etc
Metabolising enzymes:	Aminopeptidase	NA
Metabolite:	Angiotensin-III, IV,Peptides	Some fragments are active.

Details	AT-I	AT-II
Type	GPCR	GPCR
Effector Pathway	IP_3-DAG-Ca^{2+}	?
Location	Smooth muscle, neurons	
Function	Vaso constriction, ↑ NE release, ↑ Na reabsorption	↓ BP, Cell Growth
Agonists	Angiotensin	Angiotensin
Antagonists	Losartan	NA

14.   ENKEPHALIN (met- and leu-) and DYNORPHIN

Category	Chemicals/ Enzymes	Agents affecting activity
Precursors:	Proenkephalin and prodynorphin	Significantly important information is not available.
Synthesising enzymes:	Peptidases	
Metabolising enzymes:	Enkephalinase (EC 24:11) and other peptidases	
Metabolite:	Peptide fragments	

Details	μ-opoid	δ-opoid	κ-opoid
Type	GPCR	GPCR	GPCR
Effector Pathway	(↓)cAMP, (↑) K+	(↓)cAMP, (↑) K+	(↓) Ca^{2+}
Location	Pain pathway, GIT, CNS, Eye,	Pain pathway, GIT, CNS,	
Function	Analgesia, ↓ GI motility CNS depression, meiosis, euphoria	↓ GI motility, spinal analgesia	Analgesia, Dysphoria, Sedation, dependance
Agonists	DAGOL (DAMGO)	DPDPE	U69593, CI 977, dynorphin
Antagonists	Naloxone	Naltrindol	Norbinaltorphimine

15.   SUBSTANCE P (SP) AND NEUROKININS A AND B (NKA, NKB)

Category	Chemicals/ Enzymes	Agents affecting activity
Precursors:	Preprotachykinins	Significantly important information is not available.
Synthesising enzymes:	Peptidases	
Metabolising enzymes:	ACh-esterase, EC 24.11	
Metabolite:	Peptide fragments	

Details	$NK_{(1)}$	$NK_{(2)}$	$NK_{(3)}$
Type	GPCR	GPCR	GPCR
Effector Pathway	$PLC-IP_3-DAG-Ca^{2+}$	$PLC-IP_3-DAG-Ca^{2+}$	$PLC-IP_3-DAG-Ca^{2+}$
Location	Lung, bronchi, CNS	Lung, bronchi	CNS,
Function	Inflammatory action, anxiolytic, antidepressant	Inflammatory action	Anxiety
Agonists	SPOMe, GR 73632, $Sar^9Met(O_2)^{11}SP$	GR 64349	Senktide
Antagonists	GR82334, RP67580, CP-99994	L-659877, SR48968, MEN10207, GR94800 GR100679	GR138676

16. CHOLECYSTOKININ (CCK) (and GASTRIN (G))

Category	Chemicals/ Enzymes	Agents affecting activity
Precursors:	Preprocholecystokinin	Significantly important information is not available.
Synthesising enzymes:	Post-translational peptidases	
Metabolising enzymes:	Endopeptidase EC 24:11	
Metabolite:	Peptide fragments	

Details	$CCK_{(A)}$	$CCK_{(B)}$	Gastrin *
Type	GPCR	GPCR	GPCR
Effector Pathway	IP3	?	IP3
Location			
Function			
Agonists	A71378	CCK4	G17
Antagonists	Devazepide, lorglumide	L365260, PD134308	L365260

Some more neurotransmitters / hormones / signaling agents are briefly tabulated.

Signaling Agent (Abbreviation)		Receptor Type	Effector pathway	Action	Agonists	Antagonist
Antidiuretic hormone (vasopressin)	ADH	GPCR	V_1-PLc, IP_3-DAG-Ca	Vasoconstrction	Vasopressin and desmopressin	lithium and demeclocycline.
			V_2- cAMP	Vasodilation, anti diuretic		lithium
Calcitonin-gene-related peptide	CGRP	GPCR		Vasodilation		BIBN 4096 BS, hCGRP-(8-37)
Neuropeptide Y	NPY	GPCR	Ca2+	vasoconstrictor and as a cotransmitter with norepinephrine	SR120107A, BIBP 3226, BIB03304, H 409/22, SR120819A	
Neurotensin	NT	GPCR	NT1, NT2, NT3	vasodilators		SR142948A and SR48692
Oxytocin	--	GPCR G9 & G11	IP3- DAG-Ca	↑ force & frequency of uterine contraction		Atosiban
Platelet aggregating factor	PAF	GPCR	PLC-IP_3-DAG-Ca^{2+}	vasoconstriction or vasodilation	ginkgolide B,	Aspirin
Somatostatin	SS or SRIF	GPCR	Sst1		des-Ala	
			Sst2		octreotide, seglitide	
			Sst3 & Sst4		BIM23052, NNC269100	Cynamid154806
			Sst5		Sst5 C362855	BIM23056
Taurine	--	Ion Channel		Inhibitory: Cl⁻ conductance	Glycine	Strychnine

4

Regulatory Requirements in Experimental Pharmacology

During introduction we have observed that experiments can be conducted either on human beings i.e. Clinical Studies and living beings except human beings i.e. Preclinical studies. In both cases it is mandatory to seek regulatory approvals for conduction of such experiments.

Clinical Studies

In case of Clinical Studies it is mandatory to follow the guidelines issued by either national or international organization/s or even following more than one set of guideline, particularly more stringent ones, helps in submission at many countries simultaneously without going for repeated sets of studies following single set of guidelines every time. International Conference for Harmonization (ICH) guidelines are the most important to be followed if the impact of studies to be submitted to more countries since these guidelines are evolved as part of efforts to harmonize the guidelines in one set instead of having several sets of guidelines for different countries. These guidelines are available on the website of ICH i.e. www.ich.org. In India, The Indian Council of Medical Research (ICMR) has issued the guidelines which are highly acclaimed by the peers. These guidelines are available for the website of ICMR i.e. www.icmr.nic.in. Central Drugs Standard Control Organization, Ministry of Health and Family Welfare, Government of India has published "Good Clinical Practices for Clinical Research in India". The revised Schedule Y of Drugs & Cosmetics Act, 1940, amended in 2005 also deals with regulatory aspects of Clinical Trails.

In short, the guidelines for clinical studies deals with following important aspects-

Need of conduction of Clinical trials/ research, Ethical Considerations including Institutional Ethics Committee/ Institutional Review Board (IRB) etc and informed consent from the subjects/ volunteers. Several guidelines for variety of activities involving clinical studies like- Selection of participants, drug related i.e. storage condition and such other relevant information, protocol of trial, of record keeping etc.

The first step starts with formation of ethics committee.

Ethical Review Procedures

The need for ethical evaluation of research proposals has been emphasized for precaution and risk minimisation of subjects involved in clinical trials. It is mandatory that all proposals on biomedical research involving human participants should be cleared by an appropriately constituted Institutional Ethics Committee (IEC), also referred to as Institutional Review Board (IRB), Ethics Review Board (ERB) and Research Ethics Board (REB) in other countries, to safeguard the welfare and the rights of the participants. There are also independent ethics committees [IEC (Ind)] functioning outside institutions for those researchers who have no institutional attachments or work in institutions with no ethics committee. The Ethics Committees are entrusted not only with the initial review of the proposed research protocols prior to initiation of the projects but also have a continuing responsibility of regular monitoring of the approved programmes to foresee the compliance of the ethics during the period of the project. Such an ongoing review shall be in accordance with the international guidelines wherever applicable and the Standard Operating Procedures (SOP) of the WHO available at www.who.int

Basic Responsibilities

The basic responsibility of an Institutional Ethics Committee (IEC) is to ensure a competent review of all ethical aspects of the project proposals received by it in an objective manner. IECs should provide advice to the researchers on all aspects of the welfare and safety of the research participants after ensuring the scientific soundness of the proposed research through appropriate Scientific Review Committee. In institutions where this is lacking, the IEC may take up the dual responsibility of review of both, the scientific content and ethical aspects of the proposal. It is advisable to have separate Committees for each, taking care that the scientific review precedes the scrutiny for ethical issues. The scientific evaluation should ensure technical appropriateness of the proposed study. The IECs should specify in writing the authority under which the Committee is established.

Special situations

Small institutions could form alliance with other IECs or approach registered IEC (Ind). Large institutions/Universities with large number of proposals can have more than one suitably constituted IECs for different research areas for which large number of research proposals are submitted. However, the institutional policy should be same for all these IECs to safeguard the research participant's rights. A sub-committee of the main IEC may review proposals submitted by undergraduate or post-graduate students or if necessary, a committee may be separately constituted for the purpose, which will review proposals in the same manner as described above. The responsibilities of an IEC can be defined as follows:

1. To protect the dignity, rights and well being of the potential research participants.
2. To ensure that universal ethical values and international scientific standards are expressed in terms of local community values and customs.
3. To assist in the development and the education of a research community responsive to local health care requirements.

Composition

The IECs should be multidisciplinary and multisectorial in composition. Independence and competence are the two hallmarks of an IEC. The number of persons in an ethics committee should be kept fairly small (8 - 12 members). It is generally accepted that a minimum of five persons is required to form the quorum without which a decision regarding the research should not be taken. The IEC should appoint from among its members a Chairman who should be from outside the Institution and not head of the same Institution to maintain the independence of the Committee. The Member Secretary should be from the same Institution and should conduct the business of the Committee. Other members should be a mix of medical/ non-medical, scientific and non-scientific persons including lay persons to represent the differed points of view. The composition may be as follows:

1. Chairperson
2. One - two persons from basic medical science area
3. One - two clinicians from various Institutes
4. One legal expert or retired judge
5. One social scientist/ representative of non-governmental voluntary agency
6. One philosopher/ ethicist/ theologian
7. One lay person from the community
8. Member Secretary

As per revised Schedule Y of Drugs & Cosmetics Act, 1940, amended in 2005, the ethics committee approving drug trials should have in the quorum at least one representative from the following groups:

1. One basic medical scientist (preferably one pharmacologist).

2. One clinician
3. One legal expert or retired judge
4. One social scientist/ representative of non-governmental organisation/ philosopher/ ethicist/ theologian or a similar person
5. One lay person from the community.

The Ethics Committee (EC) can have as its members, individuals from other institutions or communities with adequate representation of age and gender to safeguard the interests and welfare of all sections of the community/society. If required, subject experts could be invited to offer their views, for instance, a paediatrician for paediatric conditions, a cardiologist for cardiac disorders etc. Similarly, based on the requirement of research area, for example HIV, genetic disorders etc. it is desirable to include a member from specific patient groups in the Committee.

The proposed trial should be carried out, only after approval of the Drugs Controller General of India (DCGI), as is necessary under the Schedule 'Y' of Drugs and Cosmetics Act, 1940. The investigator should also get the approval of Ethical Committee of the Institution before submitting the proposal to DCGI. All the guiding principles should be followed irrespective of whether the drug has been developed in this country or abroad or whether clinical trials have been carried out outside India or not.

Throughout the drug trials, the distinction between therapy and research should be maintained. A physician /investigator who participates in research by administering the new drug to consenting patients should ensure that the patients understand and remember that the drug is experimental and that its benefits for the condition under study are yet unproven.

Preclinical Studies

During Preclinical Research majority of the studies are conducted using various animals. The details of animals used are described elsewhere in this book. Before starting the experiments it is mandatory to have the permissions from regulating agencies for conduction of experiments. Even before it that valid permission must be obtained to keep (stock), produce (breed) and transport animals to the place of research. Although India had guidelines for animal experiments under Prevention of Cruelty to Animal Act-, the guidelines became functional after regime of Ms Maneka Gandhi, during her tenure as Minister of

"The Committee for the Purpose of Control and Supervision of Experiments on Animals", referred as CPCSEA, was empowered to form the guidelines and act as a regulatory body for the various aspects involving experimental animals. It is worthwhile to know why these guidelines and regulations are important. It is well proven fact that all biological studies show greatest variation in results. Such variation affects outcomes of many studies giving either false positive or false negative results. Thus the data acquired after utilizing several human hours and sacrificing[1] many lives (of experimental animals) becomes not only useless but may lead to wrong interpretations leading to dire consequences. The guidelines enable researchers to maintain quality of animals in such a way that there shall be minimum such variation by eliminating various stresses the animal experience due to inappropriate conditions. Details are available on Ministry of Environment and Forest, Govt of India website-

http://envfor.nic.in/divisions/awd/awd_overview.html and guidelines were also published in **Indian Journal of Pharmacology (2003; 35: 257-274).** The procedural aspects including procedure for getting CPCSEA registration (license) and proforma of Part B i.e. **Protocol form for research proposals to be submitted to the Institutional Animal Ethics Committee, for new experiments or extensions of ongoing experiments using animals other than non-human primates** are given as appendices. It is mandatory to have Institutional Animal Ethics Committee for regulating use of experimental animals and have a check on animal house facility. It constitutes with members from diverse areas of specialization with at least one from specializations like Veterinarian, Pharmacologist, Biological Scientists, social activists. The animal house in-charge can be ex-officio secretary and any one member shall be the chairman. There must be 2 biological scientists from different disciplines, a scientist from out side the institute, one scientist in charge of animal house. Once it is constituted the organization should seek license from CPCSEA for experimentation and housekeeping (establishment) of animals with or without breeding permission. At the same time CPCSEA should be requested to provide the details of its nominee on CPCSEA without presence of which the IAEC remains invalid (Gazette of India Extraordinary, 1998, Rule 13). The agenda of IAEC meeting should reach the members 30 days prior along with completely filled Part-B of Protocol (The format is enclosed as appendix 2).

Procedure of Animal Experimentation Clearance

(a) No proposal for Animal Experimentation would be entertained, unless the Animal House Facility of the concerned establishment has been approved by competent authority.

(b) The approval for experimentation on small animals will be accorded by IAEC.

(c) Approval for experimentation on Large Animals will be considered by Sub Committee on Large Animals (SCLA) on the recommendation of IAEC.

(d) The decision in the IAEC would normally be taken by consensus. If divergent views are expressed by the members these may be recorded in the minutes and a broad consensus be recorded as per understanding of the Chair. However, in case of dissent by the CPCSEA nominee, the proposal with the report of IAEC and the dissenting note of the CPCSEA nominee would be submitted to SCLA for taking a final decision.

(e) The decision in the SCLA would be taken by consensus. If divergent views are expressed by the members, these may be recorded in the minutes and a broad consensus be recorded as per understanding of the Chair.

(f) IAEC is not empowered to clear the projects above phylogenetic level higher than rodents (i.e. mice, rat, guinea pig, rabbit etc) i.e. for non-rodents (cat, dog and higher animals) the proposal should be forwarded with recommendations from IEAC to CPCSEA

Procurement of Animals

In accordance to Rule 10 of Breeding of and Experiments of Animals (control and Supervision) Rules 1998-

1. The animals must be acquired from registered breeders only or from legal sources, in case not available from registered breeders, after taking written permission from competent authority in that regard.

2. The record must be maintained of all the animals to furnish at the time of demand.

5

Experimental Animals

There are several species of animals that can be used for experimental purpose. Choice of species[1] and strains[2] is largely determined by the nature of the experiment, available facilities and the suitability for a particular type of research. The information about animals helps to understand various characteristics they possess and accordingly suitability of their use. The animals are divided in 2 ways- Small, medium and large or also as rodents and non rodents.

Mice (*Mus musculus*) - They have very acute hearing, well developed sense of smell, poor vision, small size and short generation interval[3]. They are mammals and are small, prolific and easy to maintain.

More than 3,000 genetically defined strains of laboratory mice are used for research purposes. Several characteristics have led to the increased use of mice in research. Scientists believe that mice are genetically similar to humans (at least 80 percent of DNA in mice is identical to that of humans). They are also used because of their small size, short lifespan and reproductive cycle, low maintenance in captivity, and mild manner.

Hearing is an important sense in mice and helps compensate for their poor eyesight. The poor vision of mice makes them unable to detect colour and red light is often used to observe animals during the dark cycle. Mice are highly sensitive to sound, detecting frequencies from 10-70 kHz and possibly

---

[1] **Species**- A group of related organisms having many characteristics in common and ranking below a genus which share the same heredity, are similar in morphology and behaviour, can interbreed and can produce similar offspring. They sufficiently conform to certain fixed properties and have more or less distinctive form

[2] **Strain**- An organism that is marginally different from other organisms of the same species due to genetic differences and having distinctive characteristics. e.g. Species Rat, Strain- Wistar, Sprague Dawley etc.

[3] **Generation Interval**- The interval between two successive pregnancies.

up to 100 kHz. (The human range is from 200 Hz to 16 kHz, with the most important range below 6 kHz.) The acute hearing of mice makes them highly sensitive to ultrasounds and high pitched noises inducing a stress response that has been empirically related to cannibalism of pups by their dams. The sense of taste is highly developed in mice, evident through the varied diet of wild mice. They have 16 teeth that continue to grow throughout their lifetime, so apart from eating; mice have to gnaw to prevent tooth overgrowth. There is rarely fighting among female mice groups but grouped male mice can inflict serious injuries on each other. To show their dominance over other mice in their territory, males may exhibit a behaviour termed "barbering" in which they chew distinct areas of fur, usually around the muzzle or whiskers, from subordinate mice, leaving a bald patch. The laboratory mouse is a docile animal and can be easily handled. Animals can be grouped soon after weaning usually coexists peacefully. However, some strains of mice (i.e. BALB/cJ, SJL/J, HRS/J) will begin to fight even if grouped at weaning. Breeding males that have been removed from breeding cages and caged together will usually fight. Wounds on the tail are a good sign of aggression between cage mates.

They are the primary research model used to study disorders such as cancer, AIDS, seizures, Alzheimer's disease, multiple sclerosis, and transplant rejection. There are several hundred isogenic (inbred) strains which are like immortal clones of genetically identical individuals. Each strain has its own unique characteristics and some of them are prone to diseases such as cancer, diabetes, atherosclerosis and heart disease and are used as models of similar human conditions. There are also a wide range of mutants such as obese, nude, hairless and dwarf mice. It is relatively easy to produce transgenic mice by injecting DNA into fertilized eggs and there is an extensive technology to inactivate specific genes either altogether or in specific tissues or at specific times. Genetically engineered or "transgenic" mice have selected human genes artificially introduced into their genomes that make them more susceptible to certain human diseases and conditions, such as certain types of tumours, diabetes, cancer, leprosy, tuberculosis, and even obesity. These transgenic mice are then used by researchers to study a particular ailment. Mouse DNA has been fully sequenced and several inbred strains are currently being individually sequenced. There is strong genetic linkage homology between mice and humans so that once a gene location is known in mice it's position can be predicted in humans. Mice are widely used in fundamental research, but are also used in applied research such as in toxicity testing (particularly in acute or sub-acute studies as it is smallest animal phylogenetically used for experiments) and drug development. Since it is now possible to know the genetic changes, it is also preferred for study of drugs on genetic structure like terratogenicity, mutagenicity etc. The adult mouse weighs approximately 40 grams and this small size and resulting large surface area/body weight ratio makes them susceptible to changes in environmental conditions. The core body temperature is easily affected by small changes in temperature which may modify the physiologic responses of the animal.

Rat-The Norway rat or laboratory rat *Rattus norvegicus* is a mammal of the order Rodentia is small and prolific experimental animal. Most research workers use out bred, genetically heterogeneous, rats such as Sprague-Dawley, Wistar or Long-Evans stocks. The rat genome has been fully sequenced and there are several interesting mutants like- the athymic Rowett nude and the obese "fatty" rat. The rat tends to be more widely used in applied rather than fundamental studies. It is particularly favoured for toxicological screening, physiology and behavioural studies possibly because it is larger than the mouse and exhibiting better responses. Rats have several unique biological characteristics like- acute hearing of rats makes them sensitive to ultrasounds and high pitched sounds, vision of rats is very poor and they are unable to detect colour and are blind to long-wave (red) light, the tail of the rat is the principal organ for heat exchange. There is absence of vomiting centre, gall bladder and tonsils. Since they exhibit peculiar behavioural patterns in variety of stimuli, they are widely used in psychopharmacological studies. They are almost irreplaceable for their contribution in conduction of many *in vivo* and *in vitro* experiments involving almost all systems and their organs, tissues or even cells making them important animals in most of physiological, pharmacological and toxicological studies.

Rabbit

All rabbits used for research are types of the European rabbit *Oryctolagus cuniculus*, the most common being the Californian, Florida White and New Zealand White. Rabbits are famous for their prodigious ability to reproduce. Although they share many unique characteristics, rabbits and hares differ in appearance, behaviour and ecology. Rabbits are born naked, blind, and fully dependent on the mother whereas hares are fully furred at birth, can see, and can manoeuvre on their own.

The arrangement of the lagomorph digestive system sets it apart from most other mammals. Often referred to as "hind-gut fermenters," the rabbit's digestive tract has a cecum which serves to further process food once it has passed from the stomach to the small intestine. Particles of food not broken down in the small intestine by bile and pancreatic juices enter the cecum. Here the particles stay between 2-12 hours and are further broken down by bacterial enzymes. The contents of the cecum are then deposited into the colon, where soft pellets of excreta called cecotropes are formed. Cecotropes, also referred to as "night pellets," are excreted from the colon and are sometimes re-ingested directly from the anus. The rabbit bends down to receive these pellets and swallows them whole. Ingestion of these cecotropes is vital to maintaining the rabbit's sensitive digestive tract, and once reingested, their re-digestion can take from 18 to 30 hours.

Digestive problems are common with domestic rabbits, and breeders of rabbits rapidly become familiar with a vast array of alimentary ailments. Exercise and room to move around are crucial to keeping the rabbit's digestive system functioning properly, as is access to a variety of types of roughage. In many cases, living conditions for laboratory rabbits are designed primarily with economic and husbandry concerns at the fore, with little, if any, thought given to the psychological well-being of rabbits. Rabbits should be housed with at least one other rabbit, although groups of 4-8 adult animals are ideal to mimic normal social organization, taking into account the dominance hierarchies formed by rabbits. However, in the laboratories rabbits are typically housed alone in plastic or steel cages with grid flooring, are fed a standard pellet diet, and have very little, if any, environmental enrichment. Laboratory rabbits often experience social isolation and lack of mental stimulation, conditions that often lead to abnormal behaviours associated with stress and anxiety, including incessant chewing and scratching on cage bars. Caged rabbits are also frequently denied the opportunity for normal levels of physical activity which may lead to intestinal problems and, given rabbits' light bone density, also result in osteoporosis and bone deformities

Females rarely show aggression but mature males may become increasingly aggressive if housed together, and dominance may be expressed by injuring the ears or scrotal region of subordinate males. It has been observed that in group settings, rabbit group members will stay close to those who are ill or have recently undergone surgery, which helps relieve stress and speeds healing. As an essentially nocturnal animal, rabbits are very light sensitive and need regular light and dark cycles in a lab setting. Sudden exposure to light can result in shock and even injury when the rabbit is startled. Bedding material such as straw or shredded paper provides opportunities for rabbits to exercise some control over their environment by foraging for food, building nests, digging, and maintaining their body temperature. Although pellets may be the lab rabbits' staple food, some variation should be provided such as hay and green plant material. Rabbit teeth continue to grow throughout life. Malocclusion occasionally occurs in rabbits preventing normal tooth wear resulting in severe overgrow of the teeth inhibiting normal mastication. Wooden objects for gnawing also enrich the cage environment. At minimum, cage space should allow for a normal range of motion and behaviours such as hopping, hiding and sitting up on the hind legs.

Rabbits are popular animals for research and testing primarily because they are mild-tempered and easy to handle, keep, and breed. The rabbit physiology is fairly similar to that of humans with certain exceptions like presence of atropine esterase enzyme (which metabolize atropine) in liver and plasma, absence of vasodilator nerves (responsible for exhibiting Dale's Vasomotor reversal in other animals), observation of unusual effect of histamine i.e. instead of vasodilatation it produces vasoconstriction. Rabbits also have several unique anatomical differences. The long slender ears of the albino New Zealand White breed facilitate phlebotomy procedures (use of ear vein for either administration or withdrawal of blood- Explained in chapter-4). The visibility of the peripheral vasculature in albino rabbits is advantageous to the biomedical use of this rabbit. Non-albino breeds such as the black and white Dutch belted rabbit tend to be preferred where pigmentation is required (i.e. ophthalmological research). The neutrophil of the rabbit resembles an eosinophil due to the numerous intracytoplasmic eosinophilic granules.

Rabbits are used in research for studies on variety of systems like the cardiovascular system, skin disorders, immune system, and polyclonal antibody production for use in vaccines, the most famous of which was the development of the rabies vaccine by Louis Pasteur. Polyclonal antibody production in rabbits involves injecting the animal with a chemical that is foreign to the rabbit (an immunogen) in order to stimulate a response from the immune system; this usually involves combining the immunogen with a substance that improves the immune response (known as an "adjuvant"). Rabbits are also used extensively in the study of bronchial asthma, stroke prevention treatments, cystic fibrosis, diabetes and cancer. It is official in various pharmacopoeias to use rabbit for pyrogen testing, although efforts to replace it with LAL test are on. Numerous genetic mutations have been noted in the rabbit and several inbred rabbit strains have been produced. Specific breeds of rabbit like Watanabe rabbit that normally develops coronary disease due to abnormal fat deposits in the arteries and organs, are used in the study of arteriosclerosis.

Skin and eye irritancy testing is frequently conducted on rabbits. In skin irritancy tests, areas of the rabbit's skin are shaved of fur and, in some cases, the shaved skin is abraded to remove several layers of skin cells. Then a test substance is applied to the skin. Such substances include individual chemicals or product formulations, such as cosmetics or household cleaning products. For the duration of the test the rabbit is restrained or the area may be covered to prevent licking, rubbing or other disturbances to the test area. The test area is periodically examined to assess any skin damage or penetration   into   the   bloodstream   and   any   resulting   toxic effects. Phototoxicity and photosensitization tests are similar to the skin irritancy test although the test area is exposed to light to determine what affect this will have on irritancy levels.

Rabbits are used for eye irritancy experiments because each eye has only one tear duct and test chemicals are not easily washed away. Their tear ducts are "U" shaped, and domestic rabbits sometimes require veterinary intervention if the duct becomes blocked. Since 1944 domestic rabbits have been used in the eye irritancy test known as the Draize Test which scores eye irritation from exposure to test chemicals. During the test, conscious, immobilized rabbits have test chemicals placed directly into their eyes and are left in this state up to several days to determine the irritancy level indicated by redness, ulceration, haemorrhaging, cloudiness, or blindness in the eyes. **The Draize test has been strongly criticized by scientists because it exaggerates the effects of irritants and produces results of questionable relevance to human experience.**

Guinea-pigs

The Guinea Pig, *Cavia porcellus*, is a mammal of the order Rodentia, sub-order Hystricomorpha and family Caviidae. Three basic breeds of guinea pigs exist. The English (short-haired), Peruvian (long-haired) and Absynnian which has a rosette hair pattern. Guinea pigs have several unique biological characteristics. Guinea pigs are herbivores and unlike most laboratory animals, except nonhuman primates, guinea pigs require a nutritional source of Vitamin C as their body can not produce it. Most Guinea Pigs used in research are "outbred" animals of the various breeds. The common Dunkin Hartley guinea pig is an albino outbred guinea pig of the English (short-haired) breed. Pigmented guinea pigs of all three breeds are also available. Guinea pigs are very docile and rapidly become accustomed to gentle handling, in fact guinea pigs rarely bite. Aggression between females is uncommon and is more likely to occur between males in competition for a female in estrous. Guinea pigs are easily alarmed and will often "freeze" for extended periods (30 minutes) when startled. They are important for many studies like CVS (preferred in some studies due to it's less heart rate as compared to mice and rats and better ECG recording), respiratory tract (animal with highest sensitivity to histamine), toxicological studies involving hypersensitivity reactions, hearing experiments (highly sensitive cochlea), Infectious diseases particularly tuberculosis. It is also used for bioassay of various drugs like histamine, digitalis etc. The use of guinea pigs in conduction of many *in vivo* and *in vitro* experiments involving variety of systems and their organs, tissues or even cells making them important animals in most of the physiological, pharmacological and toxicological studies

Other rodents

These include hamsters, gerbils and others. These seem to be used when no other species is found to be suitable for conducting some specific experiments.

Gerbils

Gerbils are members of the subfamily Gerbillinae (order Rodentia, family Muridae). There are about 100 species of gerbils in 14 genera. The gerbil most commonly used for research is *Meriones unguiculatus* (the Mongolian gerbil).

Gerbils are widely used in models of aural cholesteatoma, neurology (spontaneous and induced seizures), Lead neuropathy, endocrinology, genetics, hematology, infectious disease research, metabolism, reproduction, nutrition, pharmacology/toxicology, radiobiology (radioresistance) and stroke research. Additional areas of research involving gerbils have included investigations of experimental atherosclerosis and temperature regulation. Gerbils of all ages are susceptible to the human infection including Giardia duodenalis, making them good model for infection treatment.

Hamster

The Syrian hamster (*Mesocricetus auratus*) is the breed most commonly used in laboratory research, although the Chinese hamster is also popular with researchers.

Hamsters are small, docile rodents who are inactive during the day and active at night. They have large cheek pouches, which they use to transport food from the place it is gathered to the nest or den.

They are used in many experimental conditions like -Diabetes mellitus in the Chinese hamster is associated with a decrease of the pancreatic B cells. It is insulin dependent, juvenile onset and hypoinsulinemic similar to the juvenile type in man. In Syrian hamster dystrophy can be induced in various genetically modified strains. Strains susceptible for Autosomal recessive skeletal muscle degeneration, develop cardiomyopathy, cardiohypertrophy and congestive heart failure are also available. Due to variable sizes of muscle fibre, centrally located nuclei, with fatty infiltration and fibrous connective tissue replacement it is good model for physiology and pathogenesis of Duchenne's dystrophy: Cholesterol cholelithiasis (gall stones) as 90% frequency occurs in hamsters within three months, when fed diets high in simple carbohydrates and free of fat and fibre. They also provided good model for polycystic disease in an NIH hamster colony. Cardiomyopathic Syrian hamster BIO (R) 14.6 myocardial necrosis begins after one month of age in this model, leading to ventricular failure and death within one year.

Many diseases can be induced in it as an experimental animal. Hamsters are used for inhalation studies using cigarette smoke, combustion engine exhaust, and other insults with resultant cases of induced emphysema and/or interstitial fibrosis. Since the cheek pouches do not have intact lymphatic drainage, they are an ideal site for tissue transplants like tumours and grafts. They are also very good for parasitology studies and toxicology studies. They are important in radiobiology studies as the Syrian and Chinese hamsters are among the most radio-resistant animals studied.

Ferret: The ferret (*Mustela putorius furo*) share many anatomical, metabolic, and physiologic features with humans which has promoted their use as an animal model. Ferrets are used in biomedical research in a wide variety of studies including cardio-pulmonary, neurological, and gastrointestinal research. For example, ferrets are used to examine: ischemia and ion exchange in the heart muscle, pulmonary mucus secretion related to asthma or influenza, neurological changes associated with brain and spinal cord injury, and gastric infections and ulcerations. Ferrets have also been used as a model for the demonstration of medical procedures such as paediatric tracheal intubations. Use of ferrets may also be an alternative to the use of dogs, cats, or primates in some studies.

Pseudo-pregnancy can last up to 42 days. Since it has prolonged oestrus, fatal aplastic anaemia can be seen due to bone marrow depression from high levels of estrogens. Eclamptogenic toxaemia occurs prior to whelping which can be prevented with administration of raw liver. They born blind, deaf, hairless and wean at 6-7 weeks.

Their sweat glands are poorly developed. Increased heat or humidity will be stressful. They cannot digest fibre. The food transit time is 3-4 hours. It can feed on dog or cat food, supplemented with meat and vitamins. It does not have Cecum, Appendix, Prostate and Seminal vesicles. It is difficult to differentiate the small and large intestine. They are useful for CNS pharmacology studies. Their Gall bladder is contractile as in dog and man. These animals vomit readily making it necessary to fast prior to surgery. They are susceptible for stress related Gastric ulcers. They are Susceptible to avian, bovine and human TB; highly susceptible to Rabies; Heart worms (1 adult parasite can kill an adult ferret). Galvanized cages (Zinc) will kill the animals. Reye Syndrome is induced with human influenza virus, aspirin and arginine deficient diet.

CAT (*Felis catus*) - Cat can withstand prolonged anesthesia and they appear to be physiologically more akin to man than the standard laboratory rabbits and rodents makes it more preferred animal. Cancer, Parkinson's disease, genetic disorders, and auditory studies are also performed using cat. Mucopolysaccharidosis, a genetic disorder that also affects humans can be induced in cat. White cats are genetically predisposed to deafness can be used model for auditory studies.

Felines have been very widely used in acute experiments in the neurological sciences, particularly in the areas of impulse transmission, perception and the mechanisms involved in the reaction of various body systems to exposure to chemical stimuli (drugs, pollutants, etc.). They have also been extensively employed in long-term behavioral and neurological research. Cats are used as models for sleep and brain function, including sleep disorders and the effects of drugs on sleep.

In addition to other tissues, cat nictitating membrane is unique preparation for study of drug acting on ANS.

Dogs

Out of several species beagles- *Canis familaris,* are widely used in applied studies in human medicine, probably largely in toxicity testing and drug development.

It can be used for following studies-Toxicology, Pharmacology (usually - the beagle), Physiology, Surgery (usually- the Labrador, greyhound, or foxhound), Neoplasms (usually- the boxer) and Dermatology- (usually the Mexican hairless)

Beagle is preferred as it is relatively small (doesn't eat much - except for fat beagles), has short hair, is amenable to kennelling and it has good disposition

Non-human primates

About three quarters are Old-World monkeys such as Macaques; with about a quarter of them are New-World monkeys such as marmosets. A large majority of them are used in applied studies in human medicine, and in particular in toxicity testing. Much smaller numbers are used in academic research, some of which involves neuroscience and the study of diseases such as Parkinson's disease which can not always be adequately modelled in rodents.

All other species-These include sheep (0.7%), pigs (0.4%), amphibians like frog / toad (0.3%) and others (0.2%). It is difficult to generalise about why they are used. However, sheep and pigs are often used in surgical studies because of their large size and ready availability and amphibians are mostly used in fundamental developmental research. Although of great value in demonstrating simple physiological, pharmacological and toxicological concepts, experiments on frogs are no more included in curriculum at many universities in India in response to Government of India initiative to ban experimental use of frog in educational institutes. Frogs are used in experiments demonstrating physiology of nerve muscle preparation, physiology of reflex, physiology of CVS, oesophageal motility etc and effect of various drugs on it. They served as easy, economical models for many experiments which are largely replaced by experiments on mammals like rat, mice etc.

Birds

Chickens (*Gallus domesticus*) account for the vast majority of birds used in research and most of these are used in applied studies in veterinary medicine. A large proportion of these are probably embryonated eggs which are widely used to culture viruses. Recently many Pharmacologists switched to Chick tissues like ileum (brought from slaughter house) to reduce animal sacrifices at undergraduate level and minimize regulatory procedures.

Nomenclature involved for Strains of animals:

Isogenic strains

Isogenic strains include inbred strains produced by many generations of brother x sister mating, and the F1 (first generation) offspring of a cross between two inbred strains. They are like immortal clones of genetically identical individuals. The same genotype can be reproduced indefinitely, though over a period of time there may be some genetic drift due to the accumulation of new mutations. Such genetic drift is much slower than that seen in outbred stocks. Even this can be virtually eliminated using frozen embryo banks. A single individual can be genotyped at any locus, and this will serve to genotype all animals of that strain (because all are identical) so that a genetic profile can be developed for each strain. Inbred strains (but not F1 hybrids) are homozygous at all genetic loci, so will breed true, with no "hidden" recessive genes segregating within the population which may confuse experimental results. Genetic homogeneity leads to phenotypic uniformity, which means that smaller numbers of animals are needed to achieve a given level of statistical precision. Strains and individuals can usually be identified from a small sample of DNA, so that an investigator can check to see whether the animals used in a particular study were of the correct strain. Each inbred strain has a unique set of phenotypic characteristics, such as types of spontaneous disease, response to xenobiotics, behaviour etc. Some of these are valuable for a particular research project, while others would preclude the use of a particular strain from some studies. Searchable lists of inbred strains of mice and rats and their characteristics are maintained by the Jackson Laboratory. On average isogenic strains are more sensitive than outbred stocks to experimental treatments, which also increase the power of experiments which use them. They are internationally distributed, so that work can be replicated all over the world.

Mutant strains: Many mutations have arisen in mouse and, to a lesser extent, in rat colonies either spontaneously or as a result of irradiation or chemical treatment. These have been preserved for research. For example mutant athymic "nude" mice and rats have a defective cell mediated immune system and will grow human tumour xenografts. Various obese mutations have made a fundamental contribution to our understanding of obesity and metabolism.

Genetic background may influence the expression of a mutation. It is good practice to backcross them to an inbred genetic background to reduce genetic drift which may change their phenotype.

Transgenic strains: These strains are made by the incorporation of DNA from another source into the genome. This is usually done by microinjection into an early embryo. The aim is usually to get an animal to express a foreign gene, over-express a gene, or express a gene in an abnormal tissue or at an abnormal time. It is beyond the scope of this book to discuss the many uses for such strains.

"Knockout" strains: These are strains in which one or more host genes have been inactivated either altogether or in a particular tissue or at a particular time. They are widely used in fundamental research.

Outbred stocks-These are closed (usually) breeding colonies within which there is some degree of genetic variation. The amount of genetic variation depends on the previous breeding history of the particular colony. If it has been maintained in relatively small numbers (say less than 25 breeding pairs) for several generations, then it may have become relatively homogeneous (inbred). However, the extent of the genetic variation will not be known without a special genetic investigation. Investigators using species other than mouse or rats will usually have to use outbred stocks, as isogenic strains of other species are rarely available.

The biological data of commonly used animals is given in Table 5.1.

This data is aimed to be useful in many aspects- Giving information of adult age, life span of animals, feed and water pattern. This helps in knowing the basic facts about animals, the period they can be kept for study and the general care to be taken. Some other relevant factors are discussed in respective sections of next chapter which is dealing with various techniques in experimental pharmacology.

Table 5.1 General House keeping information about some laboratory animals

Parameter		MICE	RAT	HAMSTER	GERBIL	FERRET	GUINEA PIG	RABBIT	CAT	DOG
Adult body weight:	male	20-40gm	300-400 gm	85-100 gm	65-100gm	600-2000 gm	800-1200 gm	1-5 kg	2.5-3.5 kg	10-15 Kg
	female	20-40gm	250-300 gm	95-120 gm	55-85gm	550-1900 gm	700-900 gm	1.5-5.5 kg	2.5-3.6 kg	10-15 kg
Weight at Birth		1.5 gm	100 gm	2 gm	2.5-3.5 gm	6-12 gm	100 gm	100 gm	110-120 gm	250 gm
Body surface area		$10.5(\text{wt. in grams})^{2/3}$	$10.5(\text{wt. in grams})^{2/3}$	-	-	-	$9.5\ (\text{wt. in grams})^{2/3}$	-	-	-
Life span		1.5-3 years	3-4 years	1.5-3 years	3-4 years	5-9 years	4-8 years	6-12 years	12-18 years	12 years
Water consumption		15 ml/100 gm/day	10-12 ml/100 gm/day	10 ml/100 gm/day	4-7 ml/day	75-100 ml/day	10 ml/100 gm/day	5-10 ml/100 gm/day	500 ml/day	1200 ml/day
Food consumption		15 gm/100 gm/day	10 gm/100 gm/day	10-14 gm. Feed free choice	5-8 gm/day	55-75 gm/days	6 gm/100 gm/day + Vit. C	5 gm/100 gm/day	200 gm/day	18 gm/kg of complete dry diet
	Begin Dry Food Consumption	10 days	19 days	7-9 days	-	4-5 days	4-5 days	4-5 days	-	-

Contd....

Parameter		MICE	RAT	HAMSTER	GERBIL	FERRET	GUINEA PIG	RABBIT	CAT	DOG
Body Temperature	Temperature	36.5 °C	38-39°C	38 °C	37-38.5	38-40 °C	38-38.6 °C	38.5-39.5°C	38.1-39.2°C	37.9-39.9 °C
Heart rate beats/minute)	Heart Beat Adult	310-840/min	320-480 min	450/min (300-600)	360/min	250 /min	280/min (260-400)	205/minute (123-304)	110-140/min	70-160/min
	Heart Beat Newborn	328-780	250-450	-	-	-	-	-	-	-
	Breathing Rate	163/min (60-220)	85-110/min	77/min (33-127)	90/min	33-36 /minute	90/min (69-104)	51/min (38-60)	26/min	22/min
Respiratory data	O₂ Consumption	1.69 mlO$_2$/gm/hr	70-115 mlO$_2$/gm/hr	-	-	-	-	-	-	-
	Tidal volume	0.18 ml/kg	0.6-2.0 ml/kg	-	-	-	2.3-5.3 ml/kg	4-6 ml/kg	34 ml/kg	251-432 ml/kg
	Urine output	3-4 ml/100 gm B.W	5-8 ml/100 gm B.W	----------	----------	----------	4-9 ml/100 gm B.W	7-8 ml/100 gm B.W	----------	----------
	Daily faecal output	6-9 gm	9-13 gm	----------	----------	----------	15-18 gm	20-30 gm	----------	----------

71

6

Techniques for Animal Experiments-Handling, Drug Administration and other Important Techniques

Techniques in Experimental Pharmacology-

A. **Animal Related Techniques:** Animals form major part of Pharmacology experiments. It is important to know various techniques and related basic information before starting experimentations.

1. *Handling:* It is necessary to handle experimental animals in order to conduct experiments on it. If animals are not handled properly it will either not possible to conduct experiments smoothly or lead to stress in animals due rough handling making adverse impact on outcome. Initial gentle stroking of the animal followed by gradual grasping the animal will prevent startling the animal and initiating an aggressive response. Avoid approaching the animal from the front. Handling animals during the night phase can be more difficult due to increase in activity during night. While handling animals it is advisable to wear latex gloves to prevent the development of allergies due to direct contact with animal allergens. The techniques for handling rat and mice are similar i. e. pick them up with tail grasp with fingers giving support of paw. The "base" of the tail may be grasped with the thumb and forefinger. With this simple method of holding, they may be transferred to another cage or a weighing balance and can be identified, examined casually or to determine sex. For transporting short distances it may be helpful to support the rat with arm or hand while holding the tail. Rats may bite without warning, but not repeatedly and certain strains are more aggressive than others (e.g., F344 rats tend to be more aggressive than Sprague-Dawley), so care and experience are essential aspects in handling. Most important thing is that the handler must keep attention towards animal if the animal tries to rotate the head or "Spins" as it can bite the handler. Leave the animal back as soon as it is noticed that animal is turning

the head. At the same time the animal should not so firmly grasped having fear that will produce stress in animal. Rats can be also lifted by grasping the whole body with the palm over the back, with forefinger behind the head and the thumb and second finger under opposite axilla. This extends the rat's forelimbs so that they may be controlled (See figures). Holding with one hand is usually adequate for control, but the tail, rear legs or lower part of body may be held by the other hand for close control, treatment or examination. The use of both hands is often necessary for rats weighing over 350 gms. In case of heavy rats (>450 gms), rats that "spin," and when the tail is grasped more than a couple of centimetres from its base, investigators should avoid lifting by the tail as they may strip the skin from the tail. Mice can be handled in similar fashion as rats with care giving due consideration to its small size and delicate nature. Handling rabbit and guinea pig is comparatively easy. Rabbits usually do not bite but can cause scratch wounds with the hind feet. It can be grasped with the loose skin over the neck and shoulder so that the head and feet directed away from the holder. At the same time, lower part of the body must be supported by the other hand to prevent serious injury to the rabbit's back. Improper holding or frequent struggling leads to fracture of lumbar vertebrae and injury to the spinal cord. It should never be restrained or lifted by the ears. One hand should be gently placed dorsally over the thorax or ventrally under the thorax and the other hand should be used to support the animal's hindquarters. After grasping the Guinea pig it can be secured by wrapping in a towel or holding against body to lessen the frequency of struggle. It can not be held similar to rabbit grasping skin as it does not have loose skin.

2. **Transport:** The transport of animals from the source (breeder) to the laboratory requires great care to be taken. The CPCSEA has issued guidelines for the same. At the time of transport the copy of CPCSEA registration certificate should be carried by the transporter. Apart from appropriately sized and numbered boxes / cages for the given species and number of animals as prescribed in CPCSEA guidelines, air-conditioned vehicle, sufficient food and water must be provided during transport. Some time adding vegetables / fruits like- tomatoes, orange, sweet lemon serves dual purpose i.e. provides nutrition and maintains hydration. The animals must be kept in quarantine for specific days to observe changes. If found healthy, they should be transferred to their respective colonies. The quarantine is an isolated area provided inside the animal house, which do not allow the contact of newly acquired animals with existing colonies of animals. The quarantine duration varies with

animal species, strains and their physiological status i.e. for small healthy animals 7-15 days to 30-60 days for large animals. This process will also allow stabilization of animals in the new environment.

3. *Housing Conditions:* The CPCSEA has prescribed housing conditions for various experimental animals which includes room temperature, relative humidity, food and water, cage sizes, bedding material etc. The necessary details can be obtained from "CPCSEA Guidelines" which is available from various resources as mentioned in chapter 4.

4. *Sexing:* The identification of sex of animal is important aspect for many activities like selection of animals from specific sex for studies, keeping for breeding, separating male and female animals to avoid breeding etc. Identification is easier in higher animals and in lower animals it becomes easy with the advancing age. The Table 6.1 gives some information regarding identification of sex in few experimental animals. Figure also explains difference between male and female rat.

Table 6.1 Identification of sex in some experimental animals.

	Animals	**Differentiation criterion between male and Female**
1	Rat, Mice	Male and female animals can be differentiated by observing the distance between anus and genital papilla which is greater in males. After adulthood scrotum can be easily identified in male rats.
2	Rabbit, guinea pig	by causing eversion of the penis or vulva when slight pressure is applied to the external genitalia
3.	Cat, dog etc	It is easily distinguishable due presence of vagina and penis.

5. *Restraining:* Holding animal for longer time is called as restraining (literal meaning- not allowing movement). It can be done either using restraining devices or special handling methods allowing holding animal for longer time. The restraining is carefully accomplished as it can lead to stress and injury. This is required for special reasons like administration of drugs, withdrawal of fluid, Non Invasive Blood Pressure Measurement etc. one such restraining device is shown in figure.

6. *Breeding:* Common genetic categories are "random-bred" which are managed to maintain genetic diversity by mating unrelated animal;

"Inbred" which are managed to maintain genetic homozygosity by breeding siblings; "F1 hybrid" in which two inbred strains are crossbred for one generation; "knockout" in which part of the genome has been removed or inactivated; "transgenic" in which specific genetic material has been introduced into the genome of another inbred animal strain; "mutant" means which are inbred animals that have developed genetic mutations. Male: Female ratio to be kept together for mating varies species to species and usually it is 1:1 to 1:3. The Table-6.2 gives details about various breeding related information about various experimental animals. Minimum and maximum breeding age helps in planning breeding and separation of male- female animals, if breeding is not desired. Weaning period is the period after which the offspring can be separated from nursing mother, giving indication that animals can use other food (e.g. pellet). This helps in separation of male- female animals to avoid any unwarranted breeding without affecting health of grown up offsprings. Rebreed after parturition is the time taken by females to undergo another reproductive cycle after previous parturition (delivery), if kept with male.

7. **Administration**

   During experimentations various drugs are needed to be administered by any of the following routes to observe the effect of given agent. These are considered as *in vivo* administrations as whole living animal is receiving the dose of given agent. There are several routes of administration that can be divided in oral, parenteral and topical route. The details are given below-

   A. Oral (po) – administration of drug by mouth using suitable apparatus. Second form is intra-gastric in which small tube is passed through oral cavity up to stomach and drug is administered. Most of the times intragastric administration is called as gavage but sometimes oral administration is also referred as gavage. The animals' food intake may be stopped before dosing of some drugs if their absorption is affected. The duration of fasting will depend upon the feeding pattern of the species, the starting time for food restriction, physiology of the species, length of time of dosing, diet and light cycle. Large dose volumes (40 ml/kg) can overload the stomach capacity and may pass the content immediately into the small bowel and /or reflux into the oesophagus. It is recommended that for accuracy of dosing, and to avoid dosing accidents liquids are administered by gavage.

Table 6.2 Information related to Breeding of some labouratory animals

Parameter	MICE	RAT	HAMSTER	GERBIL	FERRET	GUINEA PIG	RABBIT	CAT	DOG
Male Breeding Age	50-70 days 20-35 gm	65-110 days	10-14 week 95-100 gm	70-85 days	9-12 months (700-800 gm	3-5 months 500 gm	5-6 months 4-5 kg	1 year	1-2 years
Female Breeding Age	50-60 days 20-30 gm	60-100 days	6-12 week 85-100 gm	65-85days	9-10 month	3-5 months 500 gm	6-7 months 4 kg	1 year	1-2 years
Female Estrus Cycle	4-5 days	4-5 days	4 days	4-5 days	Polyestrus	Post-partum or 16-18 days	Polyestrus	1 year	Monosterus
Gestation	17-21 days 19 days avg.	20-22 days 21 days avg	16 days 15-19 days	24-26 days	60-65 days 42 days avg	59-67 days 63 days avg	30-32 days 31 days avg	58-65 days	59-68 days Avg 63
Weaning Age	16-21 days 10-12 gm	21 days 40-50 gm	20-24 days 35 gm	21days	8 weeks 300-450 gm	10 days 250 gm	8 weeks 1.8 kg	4-6 week	4-6 week
Litter Size	1-15 10-12 avg.	8-12	6-10	3-7	5-11 8 avg	1-6 3-4 avg	1-8 8 avg	3-5	1-12 Usually 4-6
Rebreed After Parturition	Immediately	Immediately	4-6 days	-------	After weaning or next breeding season	Immediately	14-28 days	--	-------
Breeding Life Male	18 months	1 years	1 year	-------	3-4 years	5 years or longer	1-3 years	--	-------
Breeding Life Female	12-15 months 6-10 litters	1 years	10-12 month 4-5 litters	-------	2-3 years	4-5 years	1-3 years	--	-------

The housing conditions for most of the laboratory animals is similar i. e. The relative humidity should be kept in the range of 45-55%, the room temperature should be maintained in the range of $21 - 26$ °C and the light - dark cycle to be maintained at 10-12 hours/ day.

B. Parenteral-Any route other than by the alimentary canal; usually it means injected into the body. While parenteral dosing several factors must be taken in to consideration- the pH, viscosity, the dose volume used, buffering capacity, stability of the formulation before and after administration, osmolality, sterility and biocompatibility of the formulation. This is particularly important for multiple dose studies. The smallest needle size should be used taking into account the dose volume, viscosity of injection material, speed of injection and species. For non-aqueous injectables consideration must be given to time of absorption before re-dosing. There are several types depending upon site of injection and are given below-

(i) Intracerebroventricular (icv)- Into the ventricles of the brain. This requires special apparatus i.e. stereotaxic apparatus to locate ventricles beneath the skull after which the fine orifice in the skull is made with the help of small drill to administer agent in microlitre volume.

(ii) Intracerebral (ic)-Into the brain. It is done in same way as above.

(iii) Intra-arterial (ia)-Into the lumen of an artery.

(iv) Intradermal (id)-Into the dermal layer of the skin. This site is typically used for assessment of immune, inflammatory, or sensitisation response Material may be formulated with an adjuvant. Volumes of 0.05 to 0.1 ml can be used dependent upon the thickness of skin.

(v) Intramuscular (im) - Into a skeletal muscle. Intramuscular injections may be painful, because muscle fibres are necessarily placed under tension by the injected material. Sites need to be chosen to minimise the possibility of nerve damage. Sites should be rotated for multiple dose studies. A distinction needs to be made between aqueous and oily formulations (speed of absorption, oily formulations likely to remain as a depot for > 24 hours). With multiple dose studies there is a need to consider the occurrence of inflammation and its sequelae. No more than 2 intramuscular sites should be used per day.

(vi) Intraperitoneal (ip)- Into the peritoneal cavity. There is a possibility of injecting into the intestinal tract and irritant materials may cause peritonitis. The injection needle should enter at approximately $45°$ angle and before injecting the piston should be pulled back to confirm that needle has not entered in GIT or blood vessel. Drug absorption from the peritoneal cavity after the administration of the compound as a suspension is dependent on the properties of the drug particles and the vehicle, and may be absorbed into both systemic and portal circulations.

(vii) Intrathecal (it)-Into the spinal canal

(viii) Intravenous (iv) -   Into a vein. The administration can be single small volume (bolus) injection, slow small to medium volume intravenous injection, and large intravenous infusion.

Bolus injection: In most studies using the intravenous route the test substance is given over a short period, approximately 1 minute. Such relatively rapid injections require the test substance to be compatible with blood and not too viscous. When large volumes are required to be given the injection material should be warmed to body temperature. The rate of injection is an important factor in intravenous administration and it is suggested that, for rodents, the rate should not exceed 3 ml/min.

Slow intravenous injection- It can be applied due to limiting factors such as solubility or irritancy and expected clinical application of the compound. For slow intravenous injection over the course of 5 – 10 minutes a standard or butterfly needle might be used, or better still an intravenous cannula may be taped in place in a superficial vein (short term), or surgically placed some time prior to use (longer term, or multiple injections).

Continuous infusion. For similar reasons of solubility or clinical indication it may be necessary to consider continuous infusion. The volume and rate of administration will depend on the substance being given and take account of fluid therapy practice. Normally the volume administered on a single occasion will be less than 10% of the circulating blood volume over two hours. Information on circulating blood volumes is available in Table 6.6. Minimal effective restraint of animals with least stress is a key factor to consider for prolonged infusions. The total duration of an infusion is also a factor. Table 6.3 presents recommended dose rates and volumes for discontinuous (4 hour per day) and continuous (24 hour) infusion.

Table 6.3 Repeated Intravenous Infusions - Dose Volumes/Rates (and possible maximal volumes/rates)

Animal	Total Daily Volumes (ml/kg)		Rate (ml/kg/h)	
	4 Hour	24 Hour	4 Hour	24 Hour
Mouse	-	96(192)	-	4(8)
Rat	20	60(96)	5	2.5(4)
Rabbit	-	24(72)	-	1(3)
Dog	20	24(96)	5	1(4)

(-) data not available,

In some cases, two sets of figures are shown in a column. The second bracketed set of figures is the possible maximal values.

(ix) Sub-plantar- It is similar to that subcutaneous injection but it is given in the hind paw of animal to study the inflammation.

(x) Subcutaneous (sc)- Under the skin. This route is frequently used. The rate and extent of absorption depend on formulation

C. Topical-- Onto a surface, such as the skin or the eye.

Vehicles for Administration

Vehicle selection is an important consideration in all animal investigations. Vehicles themselves should offer optimal exposure but should not influence the results obtained for the compound under investigation and, as such, they should ideally be biologically inert, have no effect on the biophysical properties of the compound and have no toxic effects on the animals. If a component of the vehicle has biological effects, the dose should be limited such that these effects are minimised or not produced. Simple vehicles used to administer compounds include aqueous isotonic solutions, buffered solutions, co-solvent systems, suspensions and oils. For non-aqueous injectables consideration should be given for time of absorption before re-dosing. When administering suspensions the viscosity, pH and osmolality of the material need to be considered. The use of co-solvent systems needs careful attention since the vehicles themselves have dose limiting toxicity. Laboratories are encouraged to develop a strategy to facilitate selection of the most appropriate vehicle based on the animal study being performed and the properties of the substance under investigation.

Dose Regimes: It gives information about number of times the dose is administered in the body and the schedule if more than once a day.

(i)   Acute - Single dose.

(ii) Chronic- Repeated dosing.

    (a)   od - (Latin, *omni die*) Once daily (lit.: every day).

    (b)   bds, bd or bid- (Latin, *bis die* or *bis in die*) Twice-daily dosing.

    (c)   tds, td or tid - (Latin, *ter die* or *ter in die*) Thrice-daily dosing.

    (d)   qds or qid- (Latin, *quater in die*) Four-times-daily dosing.

    (e)   Nocte- (Latin) At night.

Administration volumes

Each site of administration has its own capacity to allow the maximum volume of administration. If the volume exceeds the limit it may lead to severe disability to animals causing stress and even painful death.

Table 6.4 Admissible Volumes of administration through various routes in some animals.

Routes of Administration	Animal Species			
	Mouse	**Rat**	**Rabbit**	**Dog**
Oral	10 (50)[1]	10 (40)	10 (15)	5 (15)
Sc	10 (40)	5 (10)	1 (2)	1 (2)
Ip	20 (80)	10 (20)	5 (20)	1 (20)
im	0.05(0.1)	0.1 (0.2)	0.25 (0.5)	0.25 (0.5)
iv (bolus)	5	5	2	2.5
Sites preferred[2]	7, 1, 5 (anaesthesia)		4	4
iv (slow inj)	-(25)	-(20)	-(10)	-(5)
Sites preferred[2]	1 (canulation),			

1. Figures given out side the bracket means ideal dose volumes for single or multiple dosing as per Good Practise Guidelines while the bracketed set of figures are the possible maximal values. Usually in cases of subcutaneous, muscular, dermal sites, administration should be limited to 2 to 3 sites per day.

2. Please refer the table 6.7. The number denotes the Serial number of the method given in the table and details of procedure are described below the table.

8. Withdrawal of blood and other fluids

Blood removal is one of the most common procedures performed on laboratory animals for obtaining haematological data for various purposes like pharmacokinetic needs (Bioavailability), observe the biomarkers for various diseases, observe changes in haematological parameters during either normal course or in disease state (natural or induced) and changes due to treatment. Normal Haematological parameters of some experimental animals are given as **Table 6.5**. It is appropriate to note that these values may not be considered as reference values as it may vary due to variety of situations like change in strain, housing condition, diet and other variables. However these values can guide the experimenter about reported values to verify the cause for drastic variation, if any.

Circulating blood volumes

The circulating blood volumes of the species commonly used in experimental Pharmacology are given in Table 6.6. These figures should help in understanding blood volume of various experimental animals and accordingly the sampling volume to be drawn.

Blood Sampling Volumes

There is little data on critical aspects of animal wellbeing after removal of blood such as heart rate, respiratory patterns, various hormonal levels, and behavioural aspects such as activities and time spent carrying them out. All these may change in response to excessive blood removal but it would require considerable effort and resource to investigate them. Single sampling (such as that required for routine toxicity studies) beyond 15% is not recommended since hypovolaemic shock may ensue if it is not done very slowly. Multiple small samples are unlikely to produce such acute effects.

Table 6.5 Information related to Hematological Data of some laboratory animals-

Parameter		MICE	RAT	HAMSTER	GERBIL	FERRET	GUINEA PIG	RABBIT	CAT	DOG
Blood Volume	-------	60-75 ml/kg	54-70ml/kg	-------	66-78ml/kg	-------	69-75ml/kg	57-65 ml/kg	47-65ml/kg	76-107ml/kg
Blood pressure	Systole	183-160	84-134	150	-------	140±35	80-94	90-130	120	95-136
	Diastole	90-110	60	100	-------	110±31	55-58	60-90	75	43-66
Blood pH	-------	7.3-7.39	7.35	7.39	7.32-7.35	7.30-7.34	7.35	7.35	7.35-7.36	7.34-7.37
RBC	-------	$7.7\text{-}12.5\times10^6/mm^3$	$7.2\text{-}9.6\times10^6/mm^3$	$4.0\text{-}10\times10^6/mm^3$	$8\text{-}9x10^6/mm^3$	$6.8\text{-}12.2x10^6/mm^3$	$4.5\text{-}7.0\times10^6/mm^3$	$4.5\text{-}7.0\times10^6/mm^3$	$5\text{-}10\times10^6/mm^3$	$5\text{-}10\times10^6/mm^3$
Hematocrit	-------	41.5ml/100ml	46 ml/100ml	49 ml/100ml	39-40/100ml	49 ml/100ml	42 ml/100ml	41.5 ml/100ml	-------	-------
Platelets	-------	$146\text{-}339\times10^3/mm^3$	$706\text{-}796\times10^3/mm^3$	$160\text{-}516\times10^3/mm^3$	$400\text{-}600x10^3/mm^3$	$766\times10^3/mm^3$	$250\text{-}850\times10^3/mm^3$	$170\text{-}1120\times10^3/mm^3$	$300\text{-}700\times10^3/mm^3$	$200\text{-}900\times10^6/mm^3$
Hb	-------	14.8 gm/100ml	14.0 gm/100ml	12.0 gm/100ml	12.6-16.2g/dl	16.5 gm/100ml	12.35 gm/100 ml	13.6 gm/100ml	8-15 gm/dl	12-18 gm/dl
Biological Values	Water	92-94 gm/100ml	92-94 gm/100ml	93-95 gm/100ml			93-95 gm/100 ml	93-95 gm/100ml		
Biological	Calcium	4.2 mEq/L	6.2 mEq/L			9.2 mEq/L	5.3 mEq/L	7.0 mEq/L		

Contd...

82

Values									
Sodium	--------	144 mEq/L	144 mEq/L	-------	150 mEq/L	145 mEq/L	140 mEq/L	-------	-------
Chloride	------	110 mEq/L	106 mEq/L	-------	116 mg/100ml	105 mEq/L	105 mEq/L	-------	-------
Phosphorus	5.6 mg/100ml	5.9 mg/100ml	-------	-------	5.9 mEq/L	5.3 mg/100ml	5.9 mg/100ml	-------	-------
Potassium	-------	5.9 mEq/L	-------	-------	5.9 mEq/L	7.4 mEq/L	5.5-6.0 mEq/L	-------	-------
Magnesium	1.3 mg/100ml	2.3 mg/100ml	1.9-2.5 mg/100 ml	-------	-------	2.3 mg/100ml	3.2-5.4 mg/100ml	-------	-------
Cholesterol	132-244(B) mg/100ml	28-76 mg/100ml	-------	90-150mg/dl	162 mg/100ml	21-43 mg/100ml	30-80 mg/100ml	2-4 mmol/L	4-7 mmol/L
Glucose	96 mg/100ml (whole blood)	56-76 mg/100ml (whole blood)	88.9-97.3 mg/100ml	50-137 mg/dl	110 mg/dl	96 mg/100ml (whole blood	145 mg/100ml (whole blood)	81-108 mg/dl	54-99 mg/dl
Serum Protein	174 gm/100ml (white blood)	6.3 gm/100ml	-------	4.3-12.5g/dl	6.0 gm/100ml	5.4 gm/100ml	7.2 gm/100ml	6-7.5 gm/dl	6-7.5 gm/dl
Albumin	3.4 gm/100ml	3.4-4.3 gm/100ml	-------	1.8-5.5g/dl	3.2 gm/100ml	3.2 gm/100ml	4.6 gm/100ml	2.5-4 gm/dl	3-4 gm/dl
Globulin	0.6 gm/100ml	1.8-2.5 gm/100ml	-------	1.2-6g/dl	2.6 gm/100ml	2.2 gm/100ml	2.7 gm/100ml	2.5-3.8 gm/dl	2.4-3.7 gm/dl
Creatinine	0.3-1 mg/dl	0.2-0.8 mg/dl	0.91-0.99 mg/dl	0.6-1.4 mg/dl	0.4-0.9 mg/dl	0.6-2.2 mg/dl	0.8-1.8 mg/dl	<180μm ol/1	<128 μmol/l

Contd...

83

		12-28	15-21	12-25	-----	-----	9-31.5	17-23.5	3.5-8	3.5-7
Hematological Values	Urea nitrogen	12-28	15-21	12-25	-----	-----	9-31.5	17-23.5	3.5-8	3.5-7
	Whole Blood Vol	78 ml/kg	58 ml/kg	85 ml/kg	66-78ml/kg	-----	75 ml/kg	60 ml/kg	-----	-----
	Clotting Time	14 sec.	20 sec.	143 sec.	-----	-----	60 sec.	60-360 sec.	-----	-----
	RBC Life Span	20-30 days	45-68 days	-----	-----	-----	-----	45-70 days	-----	-----
	RBC Diameter	6.6 microns	6.8 microns	-----	-----	6.1 microns	7.1 microns	7.0 microns	-----	-----
	RBC Rate of Sedimentation	-----	0.7-1.8 mm/hr	2 mm/hr	-----	-----	0.5-1.5 mm/hr	2 mm/hr	-----	-----
Total and Differential White Blood Cell Counts	Leucocytes	$8.0\times 10^3/mm^3$	$14.0\times 10^3/mm^3$	$3\text{-}11\times10^3/mm^3$	$7\text{-}15\times10^3/mm$	$9.2\times 10^3/mm^3$	$10.0\times 10^3/mm^3$	$9.0\times 10^3/mm^3$	$5.5\text{-}19.5\times 10^3/mm^3$	$6\text{-}17\times 10^3/mm^3$
	Neutrophils	$2.0\times 10^3/mm^3$	$3.1\times 10^3/mm^3$	10-13%	5-34 %	49 %	$4.2\times 10^3/mm^3$	$4.1\times 10^3/mm^3$	35-75%	60-70%
	Eosinophils	$0.18\times 10^3/mm^3$	$0.3\times 10^3/mm^3$	0-4.5%	0-4 %	3.4 %	$0.4\times 10^3/mm^3$	$0.18\times 10^3/mm^3$	2-12%	2-10%
	Basophils	$0.05\times 10^3/mm^3$	$0.10\times 10^3/mm^3$	0-1%	0-1 %	0.4 %	$0.07\times 10^3/mm^3$	$0.45\times 10^3/mm^3$	Rare	Rare
	Lymphocytes	$5.5\times 10^3/mm^3$	$10.0\times 10^3/mm^3$	50-95%	60-95 %	45 %	$4.9\times 10^3/mm^3$	$3.5\times 10^3/mm^3$	20-55%	12-30%
	Monocytes	$0.30\times 10^3/mm^3$	$0.30\times 10^3/mm^3$	0-3%	0-3 %	1.15%	$0.43\times 10^3/mm^3$	$0.73\times 10^3/mm^3$	1-4%	3-10%

The following guide for limit volumes and adequate recovery period takes into account the stress of multiple sampling in addition to other procedures in assessing overall severity. The table 6.6 addresses both single and multiple sampling regimes. Additional recovery time is proposed for animals on toxicity studies since a critical evaluation of haematological parameters is required in such studies.

Limit volumes and recovery periods- Whenever blood is withdrawn it causes impact on physiology of animal. Usually when 7.5 %, 10%, 15% blood of total circulatory volume in the body is withdrawn whether as single sampling or multiple sampling in 24 hours it takes 1, 2 and 4 weeks respectively to recover from the impact.

Table 6.6 Blood volumes and Guidelines for withdrawal of blood in some experimental animals.

Species	Body weight range (g)	Blood volume (ml/kg)	Total blood volume (TBV), in normal adult (ml)	Blood Volume Safely withdrawn from single bleed (ml)	Terminal Bleeding volume (ml)
Mouse	18 - 40	58.5	M 1.5 - 2.4, F 1.0 - 2.4	0.1 - 0.2	M 0.8 - 1.4 F 0.6 - 1.4
Rat	250 - 500	54 - 70	M 29 - 33 F 16 - 19	M 2.9 - 3.3, F 1.6 - 1.9	M 13 - 15 F 7.5 - 9
Hamster	85-150	78	M 6.3 - 9.7, F 7.1 - 11.2	M 0.6 - 0.9, F 0.7 - 1.1	M 2.9 - 4.5 F 3.3 - 5.2
Gerbil	55 - 100	66 - 78	M 4.5 - 7 F 3.8 - 6	M 0.4 - 0.7, F 0.4 - 0.6	M 2.2 - 3.5 F 1.9 - 2.9
Guinea pig	700 - 1200	69 - 75	M 59 - 84 F 48 - 63	M 6 - 8 F 5 - 6	M 29 - 42 F 24 - 31
Rabbit	1000 - 6000	57 - 65	58.5	5 - 50	31 - 310
Ferret	600- 2000	70	42 - 140	4 - 14	21 - 70
Dog	7000-10000	70 - 110	900 - 1170	90 - 110	-
Cat	-	47 - 65	140 - 200	14 - 20	-

M-Male, F-Female

Table 6.7 Summary of the methods of blood sampling single or multiple times along with some important features of each site.

No	ROUTE/VEIN	General Anaesthesia	Tissue damage[1]	Repeat bleeds	Volume[2]	Recommended site for single sampling in species	Recommended site for multiple sampling in species
1	Jugular	no	low	yes	+++	rat, dog, rabbit	Rabbit, rat, Dog
2	Cephalic	no	low	yes	+++	macaque, dog	Dog, Macaque
3	Saphenous/lateral tarsal	no	low	yes	++(+)	mouse/rat marmoset /macaque, dog	Mouse, Rat, Dog, Macaque, Marmoset
4	Marginal ear	no (local)	low	yes	++ +	rabbit minipig	Rabbit
5	Femoral	no	low	yes	+++	marmoset/macaque	Macaque, Marmoset
6	Sub-lingual	yes	low	yes	+++	rat	Rat
7	Lateral tail	no	low	yes	++(+) +	rat mouse/marmoset	Mouse, Rat
8	Central ear artery	no (local)	low	yes	+++	rabbit	Rabbit
9	Cranial vena cava	no	low	yes	+++	minipig	Minipig
10	Tail tip amputation (<1 to 3mm)	yes	mod	limited	+	mouse/rat	
11	Retrobulbar plexus	yes	mod/high	yes	+++	mouse/rat	
12	Cardiac[3]	yes	mod	no	+++	mouse/rat/rabbit	

Sampling sites: The blood may have to be withdrawn once or for multiple times. The site (blood vessel) shall be selected accordingly. Following table summarises with the recommended ones for single and repeated blood.

1. The potential for tissue damage is based on the likelihood of occurring the incidence and the severity of any sequel like damage to tissue etc.
2. + indicate minimum while + + + indicate maximum volume of blood that can be withdrawn fro the site,
3. Only carried out as terminal procedure under general anaesthesia

It is important to note that samples taken from different sites may show differences in clinical pathology values and have implications for historical databases.

For the more traditional routes, a description of the methodology can be obtained from the standard literature. However, other methods require a special mention and have been reviewed below:

Lateral tarsal (saphenous) vein: This technique has been used in many laboratory animals including rats, mice, hamster, gerbil, guinea pig, ferret, mink and larger animals for withdrawal of blood volumes up to 5% of circulating blood volume. It does not require an anaesthetic and so is particularly suitable for repeated blood sampling as in pharmacokinetic studies. The saphenous vein is on the lateral aspect of the tarsal joint (ankle joint) and is easier to see when the fur is shaved and the area wiped with alcohol. The animal is placed in a suitable restrainer, the hind leg is extended and the vein is raised by gentle pressure above the joint. The vessel punctured using the smallest gauge needle that enables sufficiently rapid blood withdrawal without haemolysis (e.g. 25g to 27g for rats and mice). After blood has been collected, pressure over the site is sufficient to stop further bleeding. Removal of the scab will enable serial sampling. It is best method as no anaesthesia is required and no complications are known except persistent bleeding in few cases.

Marginal ear vein/central ear artery: Blood sampling from marginal ear vein is a common practise in case of rabbits and guinea-pigs

Sublingual vein: This technique is easy to perform in rats and is suitable for the removal of 0.2 to 1ml of blood at frequent intervals. Rats are anaesthetised and held in a supine position by one person. A second person gently pulls out the tongue with a cotton-tipped applicator stick and grasps it with thumb and forefinger and one of the sublingual veins (there is one each side of the midline) is punctured with a 23 – 25g hypodermic needle as near to the tip of the tongue as possible. The rat is turned over to allow blood to drip into a tube and after the requisite volume of blood has been obtained, the compression at the scruff of the neck is released and the animal placed in a supine position. The tongue is again extended in order to stem the flow of blood with a dry cotton-tipped applicator stick; usually there is no need to use any haemostatic agent. Rats do not show any significant differences in food or water consumption or bodyweight. It is believed to be better that retroorbital blood withdrawal. However, less blood volume to be removed and necessary repeated anaesthesia are the limiting factors.

Lateral tail vein: This route yield smaller blood volumes (0.1 to 0.15ml in mice, up to 2 ml in warmed rats) as compared to Saphenous vein. Blood is removed either by syringe/needle or stab puncture of a lateral tail vein. Anaesthesia is unnecessary which makes this route particularly suited for repeated blood sampling and administration. Vasodilatation may be necessary to promote bleeding and can be caused by exposing an animal to 37°C for 5 to 8 minutes or by local warming of the tail using warm water. The tip of tail should be used as vein is clear and the proximal parts can be used during next administrations or in case the first attempt is not successful. Please see photograph

Amputation of the tail tip: This technique is commonly used in rats and mice, with sample volumes of 0.1 to 0.2ml being obtained. Amputation should be restricted to the tail tip 0.5 to 1mm should be adequate, and over time a maximum of 5mm being removed) and repeat bleeding is feasible in the short term by removing the clot. Serial amputations resulting in a significant shortening of the tail (i.e. >5mm) are not acceptable. The technique may not be suitable for older animals. Anaesthesia is recommended.

Cardiac puncture: This should always be carried out under general anaesthesia and in the past it has been used with recovery in small rodents due to the lack of alternative routes. However, other methods are now available and because of potentially painful and fatal sequelae such as pericardial bleeding and cardiac tamponade, this technique should only be used for terminal bleeds.

Retrobulbar plexus: The retrobulbar route is the most commonly used method by researchers. However, it causes severe adverse impact on animal. Therefore other methods have been developed which meet the scientific requirements and also improve the welfare of the animals. Bleeding from this plexus should always be carried out under general anaesthesia in all species and anaesthesia is a requirement in some national regulations. Please see photograph.

There are several serious potential adverse effects:

- any pressure required to control persistent bleeding (i.e. pressing the eye) or pressure due to haematoma can lead to keratitis, corneal ulceration, pannus formation, rupture of the globe and micro-ophthalmia all these are painful for the animal;

- deficits in vision and even blindness due to damage to the optic nerve and other intra-orbital structures;
- fracture of the fragile bones of the orbit and neural damage by the micro-pipette; and
- penetration of the eye globe itself with a loss of vitreous humour.

Many of these unwanted sequelae may stay undetected being located deep within the orbit.

To summarise-

- sampling by cardiac routes is only carried out as a terminal procedure under general anaesthesia;
- retrobulbar sampling with recovery should only be used when other routes are not practical; and
- recommended routes for bleeding are the lateral tail vein, the sublingual vein and the lateral tarsal vein for all rodents, and the marginal ear vein, central ear artery and the jugular vein for rabbits.

Cannulation

This is an important technique for repeated bleeds and administration. Temporary cannulae such as butterfly needles and over-the-needle cannulae can be used in the short-term (working day), whereas for long-term use, surgical implantation of biocompatible cannulae is required. Following factors govern the use-

- Surgical skills are essential and it must be done sterilely for good long term performance and to avoid complications such as infection. Clotting frequently occurs and may prevent both blood removal and prolonged infusion of substances.
- It may be necessary to restrain an animal or to separate it from its peers in order to prevent removal or biting of the attached external cannulae and that is why a subcutaneous venous access port is preferred for long-term use.
- After long-term cannulation penetration of the vessel can occur and an animal may also outgrow its cannula.

9. Anaesthesia

Not only to follow guidelines of CPCSEA but also for ethical reasons agents like- sedatives, analgesics and anaesthetics should be used to control pain or distress to animal under experiment unless contrary to the achievement of the results of study. The care must be exercised for selecting anaesthetic agents as they generally affect cardiovascular, respiratory and thermoregulatory mechanism in addition to central nervous system.

Local or general anaesthesia may be used, depending on the type of surgical procedure. Local anaesthetics are used to block the nerve supply to a limited area and are used only for minor and rapid procedures. This should be carried out under expert supervision for regional infiltration of surgical site, nerve blocks and for epidural and spinal anaesthesia. A number of general anaesthetic agents are used in the form of inhalants like many gaseous anaesthetics, intravenous or intra-muscular injections such as barbiturates. Species characteristics and variation must be kept in mind while using an anaesthetic. Side-effects such as excessive salivation, convulsions, excitement and disorientation should be suitably prevented and controlled. The animal should remain under veterinary care till it completely recovers from anaesthesia and postoperative stress. In general, there are two different routes to induce general anaesthesia: (i) injection and (ii) inhalation anaesthesia. Sometimes combinations of both routes are used. The decision for one or the other route depends on the animal species, the purpose of the study and the necessity of control during anaesthesia.

Injection: By using this route of anaesthesia the narcotic compound is dissolved in a liquid. The route of administration can be intravenous, intramuscular, subcutaneous or intra-peritoneal. The most frequently used compounds are mentioned below in **Table 6.8.**

Inhalation

Inhalation anaesthesia is more common for the bigger laboratory animals such as dogs, cats, sheep, goats and monkeys and plays only a minor role for small laboratory animals like rodents. It can be used in rodents too for short durations as in case of blood withdrawal etc. as shown in a photograph at the end of this chapter. The advantages of this method are the possibilities of controlling exactly the depth of anaesthesia and of fast management of complications.

Termination of anaesthesia

Inhalation anaesthesia can be stopped by removing the supply of evaporated compounds. To hasten the elimination of anaesthetic compounds, the concentration of oxygen in the system can be increased for a period of five min. The elimination of injected compounds is difficult to monitor and control. It may be possible to accelerate metabolism of the anaesthetic by using agents which stimulate metabolism in the liver and excretion by the kidney.

It is very important to check the body temperature of the animal during and after anaesthesia. In cases of low body temperature the use of heating lamps or pads is necessary. During anaesthesia it might be necessary to stimulate respiration or circulation. Stimulatory agents for respiration are doxapram, pentamethylentetrazole, nikethamide, methetarimide, lobeline or micoren. Stimulatory agents for circulation are adrenaline, dobutamine, effortil, dopamine and ephedrine. The application of pure oxygen via a mask is also recommended during inhalation anaesthesia. Antidotes to morphine and its derivatives are morphine-antagonists like naloxone. Yohimbine is an antagonist of xylazine. The antidote for diazepam is flumazenil. There are no direct antagonists for ketamine and barbiturates.

Table 6.8 Anaesthesia in some experimental animals (values are in mg/kg)

Species	Short anaesthesia	Medium anaesthesia	Long anaesthesia
Mouse	Inhalation (Isoflurane) or Alfentanyle (0.02-0.03) + Etomidate (1.5-2.5)	Xylazine (4-6) or Diazepam (2-3) + Ketamine (100) or Pentobarbitone (50)	Xylazine (14-17) + Ketamine (100)
Rat	Inhalation (Isoflurane) or Alfentanyle (0.02-0.03) + Etomidate (1.5-2.5)	Xylazine (4-6) or Diazepam (2-3) + Ketamine (100) or Pentobarbitone (50)	Xylazine (14-17) + Ketamine (100) or Urethane (1200-1600)
Hamster	Inhalation (Isoflurane or Ether)	Xylazine (4-6) or Diazepam (2-3) + Ketamine (100) or Pentobarbitone (30-40)	Xylazine (10) + Ketamine (200)
Guinea Pig	Inhalation (Isoflurane)	Xylazine (2-3) + Ketamine (70- 85)	Xylazine (4-6) or Diazepam (2-3) + Ketamine (100) or Pentobarbitone (30) + Chloralhydrate (300)
Rabbit	Inhalation (Isoflurane)	Xylazine (4-6) or Diazepam (2-3) + Ketamine (70-100)	Xylazine (4-6) or Diazepam (2-3) + Ketamine (100) or Pentobarbitone (30) + Chloralhydrate (300)
Cat	Acetylpromazine (0.5–1 i.v./i.m.) or Xylazine (2 i.m.) or Propionylpromazine (0.5–1 i.v.)	Xylazine (2) + Ketamine (10) or Ketamine (5 i.v.) or Inhalation (Isoflurane)	Pentobarbitone (30-45 i.v./i.p.)

Contd...

Species	Short anaesthesia	Medium anaesthesia	Long anaesthesia
Dog	Thiopental (17 i.v.) or Metomidate (4) + Fentanyl (0.005) or Alfentanil (0.03) + Etomidat (1) or Inhalation/ Intubation (Isoflurane)	Xylazine (2) + Methadone (1) or Xylazine (2) + Ketamine (10) or combined with Diazepam (0.6 i.m.) or Methadone (1) + Propionylpromazine (0.5) or Methadone (1) + Acetylpromazine (0.5)	Pentobarbitone (30 i.v.) or Xylazine (2) + Ketamine (15) or Inhalation (Isoflurane)

Usual routes of administration for Xylazine (im), Diazepam (im), Ketamine (im or ip), Pentobarbitone (ip), Chloral hydrate (iv) are as given in bracket except those mentioned above. i.m. = intramuscular, i.v. = intravenous, i.p. = intraperitoneal, s.c. = subcutaneous.

Atropine (0.02 - 0.05 mg/kg) by s/c or i/m or i/v routes may be administered to reduce salivary and bronchial secretions and protect heart from vagal inhibition in most of the species, given prior to anaesthesia. In some case sedatives like diazepam can be administered.

10. *Euthanasia:* The method for humane and painless (gentle death) sacrifice[1] of animals to avoid suffering after experimentation is called as Euthanasia. Animals may have to be sacrificed in biomedical laboratories (i) at the end of an *in vivo* experiment, (ii) during experiments where sacrifice of the animals is not part of the study but must be done when pain, distress and suffering exceed acceptable levels or if it is likely for the animal to remain in pain or distress after cessation of the experiment, and (iii) to provide biological material for *in vitro* studies. The procedure should be carried out quickly and painlessly in such a way that animals should be free from fear or anxiety. For accepting a euthanasia method as humane it should have an initial depressive action on the central nervous system for immediate insensitivity to pain. The euthanasia method must always meet the following requirements:

(a)   Minimum physiological and psychological disturbances

(b)   Compatibility with the purpose of study and minimum emotional effect on the operator.

(c)   Death, without causing anxiety, pain or distress with minimum time lag phase.

---

[1] Sacrifice- The death of animal at the hands of experimenter during or after experiments is referred to as sacrifice instead of killing as it is for the noble cause of science and not for any other different purpose.

(d)   The method should be reliable, reproducible and irreversible

(e)   Location should be separate from animal rooms and free from environmental contaminants.

The euthanasia warrants extreme care as distress vocalization and release of certain odours or pheromones by a frightened animal may cause anxiety in other animals housed nearby. It must be noted that many vocalisations of animals are in a range of frequencies which are out of the human hearing range. Therefore, other animals should not be present during euthanasia of animals, especially of their own species. If possible, an animal should not be killed in a room where other animals are housed, in particular in case of a bloody method of euthanasia, e.g. decapitation.

The person performing euthanasia is the most relevant factor during sacrificing an animal in order to cause a minimum of pain, fear and distress. A suitable method of euthanasia can be extremely harmful to the animal if it is badly performed. All persons performing euthanasia must be well trained, demonstrate professionalism and should be sensitive to the value of animal life.

Methods for euthanasia of laboratory animals can be separated into physical and chemical methods.

Physical methods recommended for euthanasia of laboratory animals-Physical methods are stunning (concussion, electrical stunning, and stunning with a captive bolt), cervical dislocation, decapitation, and microwave irradiation. The different methods of stunning as well as cervical dislocation cause a rapid loss of consciousness which must be followed immediately by a method to force and guarantee death of the animal. Concussion may be sufficient in smaller animals, e.g. rodents, to achieve unconsciousness and is performed by a blow to the head. Cervical dislocation destroys the brainstem but the large vessels to the brain are often intact. All these methods have to be followed immediately by an act to force and guarantee death, e.g. exsanguination, removal of the heart or destruction of the brain. During the decapitation process the head is separated from the neck which causes an immediate interruption of the blood circulation to the brain and a fall in blood pressure in the brain with subsequent loss of consciousness. This is valid only for warm-blooded animals. In cold-blooded vertebrates it is recommended to stun the animals prior to decapitation due to their higher resistance against anoxia. For decapitation of smaller laboratory animals specific guillotines have been developed.

Chemical agents recommended for euthanasia of laboratory animals-Many chemicals can cause death due to their toxicity, but only a few are recommended for euthanasia. The most suitable chemicals for euthanasia are certain anaesthetics in overdose. In this case, the anaesthetic agent causes unconsciousness, followed by death. Carbon dioxide at high concentrations of 80 to 100% causes unconsciousness within a few seconds. Injectable anaesthetics, predominantly barbiturates such as sodium pentobarbitone, are the most widely used and the most appropriate agents for euthanasia for most animals. Three times the anaesthetic dose causes generally rapid unconsciousness and death. As far as possible intravenous injections should be preferred over other routes as it is most rapid method.

Methods and agents not to be used for euthanasia of laboratory animals

There are many methods which should not be used even though can cause death of animal. Physical methods not to be used for euthanasia are exsanguination, rapid freezing, pithing, decompression, hyperthermia, hypothermia, asphyxia, drowning and strangulation. Some chemicals are not recommended for euthanasia because they are extremely noxious and dangerous to the persons in laboratory. Chemicals not to be used are carbon monoxide, nitrogen, nitrous oxide, cyclopropane, chloroform, trichloroethylene, hydrogen cyanide, magnesium sulphate, potassium chloride, nicotine, strychnine, chloral hydrate, and ethanol. Neuromuscular blocking agents such as curare, succinylcholine or suxamethonium are also not preferred as they do not cause rapid unconsciousness prior to death. Ketamine is unsuitable for euthanasia although it is very good anaesthetic, due to its wide therapeutic safety margin for most animal species. However, non-acceptable methods of euthanasia can be used in anaesthetized animals or animals rendered insensible using a recommended method e.g. exsanguination, rapid freezing, and pithing.

Methods Not Preferable for any species of animals-

1. Physical methods- Decompression and Stunning (stunning becomes a painful process requiring several blows if not performed by an expert)

2. Inhalation of gases -Nitrogen Flushing and Argon Flushing

3. Drug administration - Curariform drugs, Strychnine, Nicotine sulphate, Paraquat, Magnesium sulphate, Dichlorvos, Potassium chloride, Air Embolism

Table 6.9 Recommended methods for euthanasia for specific animal species

Species	Mouse	Rat	Hamster	G. pig	Rabbit	Cat	Dog	Monkey
1. Physical Methods								
Electrocution	NP	NP	NP	NP	NP	NP	NP	NP
Exsanguination	P	P	P	P	P	P	NP	NP
Decapitation (for analysis of stress)	P	P	NP	NP	NP	NP	NP	NP
Cervical dislocation	P	P	P	NP	NP	NP	NP	NP
2. Chemical Methods								
(b) Inhalation of gases								
Carbon monoxide	P	P	P	P	P	P	P	P
Carbon dioxide	P	P	P	P	P	P	NP	NP
Carbon dioxide plus	P	P	P	P	P	P	NP	NP
chloroform /halothane	P	P	P	P	P	P	P	P
(c) Drug administration								
Barbiturate overdose (route)	P(IP)	P(IP)	P(IP)	P(IP)	P(IV, IP)	P(IV, IP)	P(IV, IP)	P(IV, IP)
Chloral hydrate overdose (route)	NP	NP	NP	P (IV)	P (IV)	P (IV)	P (IV)	
Ketamine overdose (route)	P(IM/IP)	P(IM/IP)	P(IM/IP)	P(IM/IP)	P(IM/IV)	P(IM/IV)	P(IM/IV)	P(IM/IV)
Sodium pentothol [overdose (route)]	IP	IP	IP	IV	IV IV	IV	IV	IV

im = intramuscular, iv = intravenous, ip = intraperitoneal. Note- subcutaneous route is not suitable as it has very slow onset and long lasting effect.

(P – Preferable Methods for the given species of animals indicated NP - Not Preferred)

11.   ***Disposal***: After sacrifice the body of animal should be disposed with respect and utmost care so that it is not taken away by stray animals, birds etc. The careless disposal not only leads to spread of diseases but also it is unethical to throw the Caracas of "Sacrificed" animal. There are various ways proposed for it – deep burial in the ground and use of incinerator to burn the animal.

B. Instrument Related Techniques

It is important to use instruments carefully and as prescribed in the manual. Details of some of the instruments specific techniques are given in the Chapter- 10 dealing with instruments. Generally following precaution to be taken-

Where ever available the instruments must be operated as per operation manual provided or as per expert's direction. The instrument must be calibrated using standard available for the given parameter before either start of experiment or as prescribed in the manual / experts. It is important to verify the functioning of all the parts before starting the experiment. Most of the equipments or their out put are affected during voltage fluctuations as evident by damage to instrument or unjustified responses during the experiments. This can be avoided by using suitable voltage stabilizers.

C. Other Preparations

The required solutions and their dilutions must be prepared as per standard formulae and method. The details about various considerations are dealt with in chapter 2- Understanding Basics.

D. Personnel

The experimenters must be acquainted rather trained in various aspects of conduction of experiments like selection of appropriate model/s, parameter/s and their feasibility in the given set up. The proficiency, experience and strong fundamentals of the experimenter/s shall be the key components in successful outcome of experiments.

E. Data Analyses

Use of appropriate statistical techniques from the conceptual phase (making hypothesis) to planning i.e. making protocol till data analyses after final results forms important segment in experimental pharmacology. The use and appropriateness of various statistical techniques are described in chapters- Humane, CAL and Computers

All these techniques, as described above, form important pillars of experimental pharmacology and their knowledge is must for a Pharmacologist to minimize errors and variations in the out come of any pharmacological study.

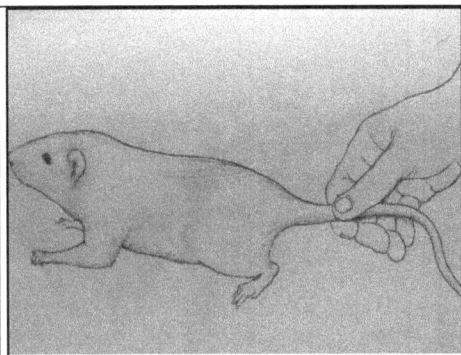

Holding rat / mouse using tail and handling for short period like transfer from cage etc.

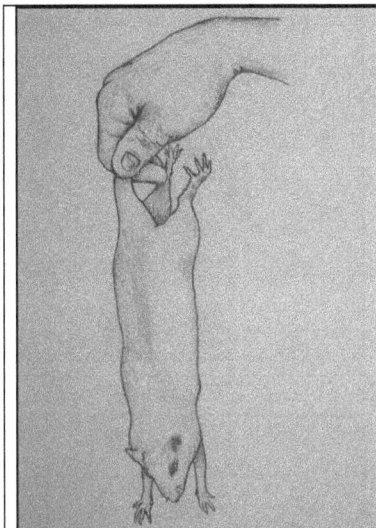

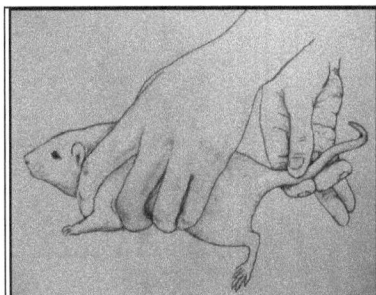

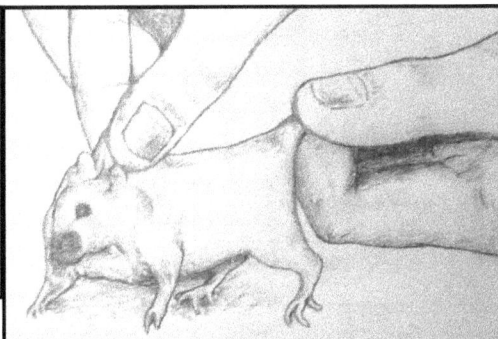

Holding rat / mouse for more time and for administration either by oral, intramuscular or intra peritoneal route.

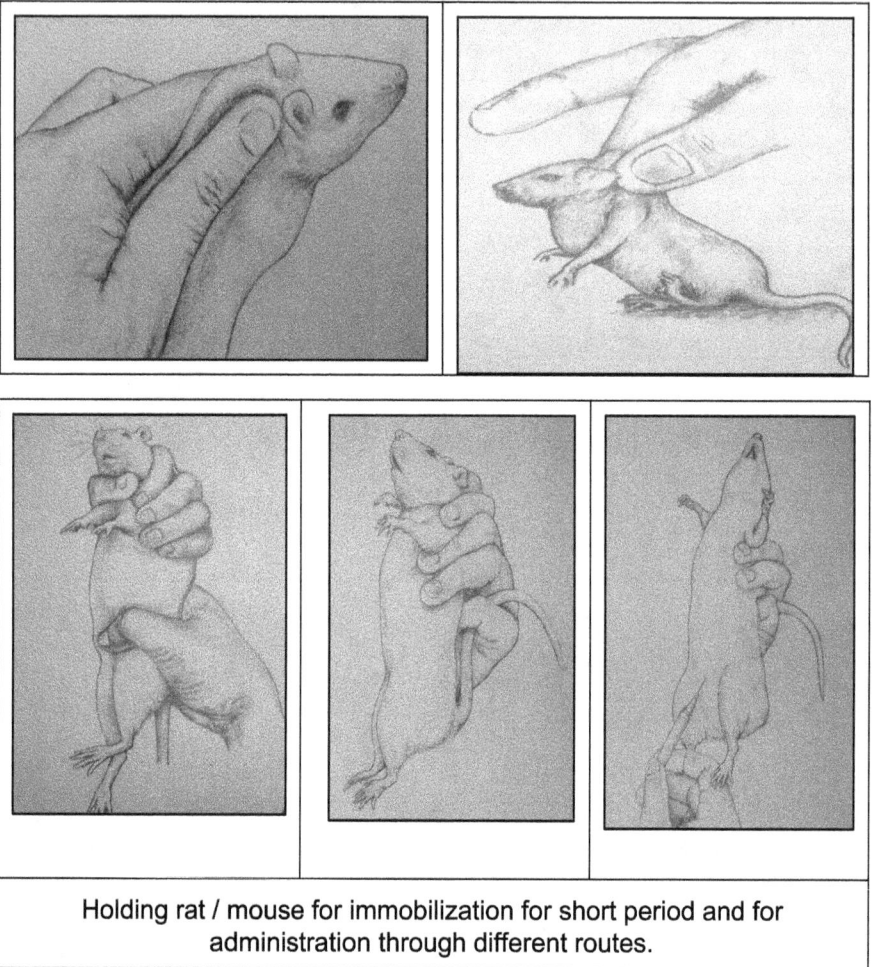

Holding rat / mouse for immobilization for short period and for administration through different routes.

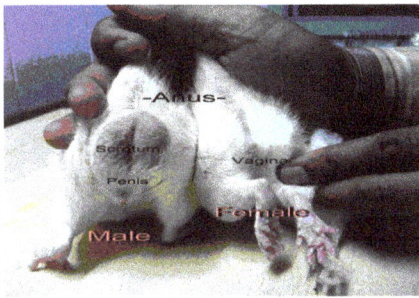

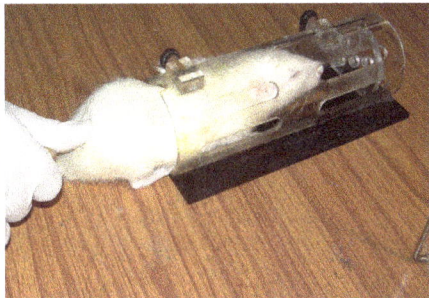

| Identification of male and female animals respectively by anogenital distance | Use of restrainer for holding rat / mouse for long time (NIBP measurement) and iv administration etc |

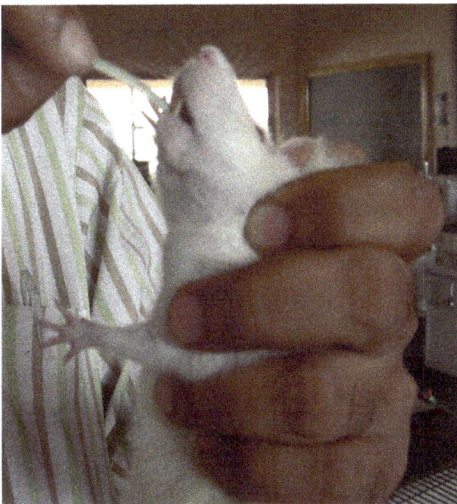

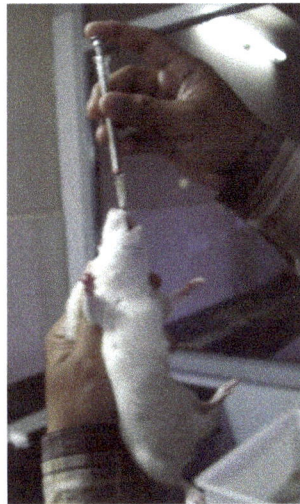

Holding rat / mice for intra gastric and oral administration (gavage). Figure shows insertion of Infant Ryle's tube ithorugh oral cavity for intra hastric administration

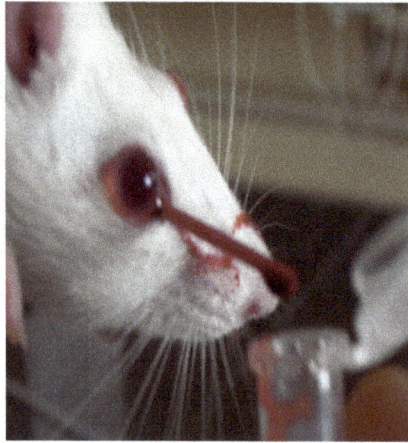

Blood Withdrawal from retro orbital sinus of rat (under mild ether anesthesia). Use short, less fragile capillary from smooth end.

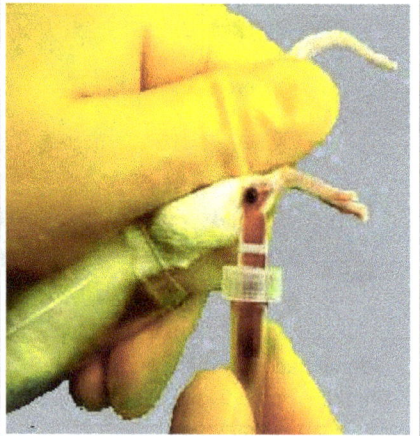

Blood Withdrawal from saphenious vein of mouse. The mouse is placed in tube like restrainer and vein is exposed with removal of hairs, vein is punctured with needle.

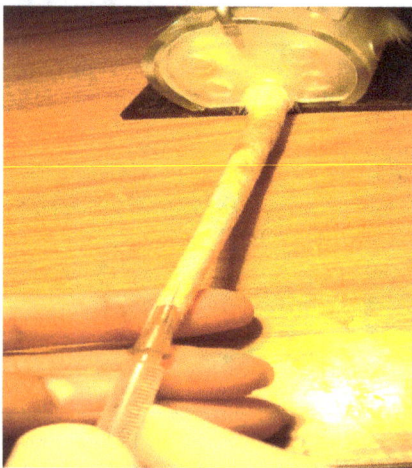

Iv injection in tail vein. Locate vein close to tip of tail to avoid leakage if subsequent injections are needed and for better insertion of needle.

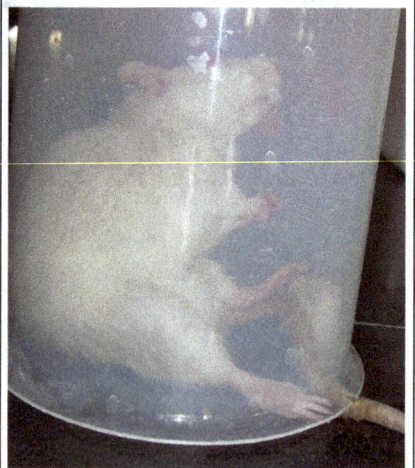

Anesthesia using volatile anesthetic (ether / chloroform). Cotton wool soaked with agent is placed in transparent box / beaker etc and observed till anesthesia is achieved.

7

Humane Approaches in Pharmacology Experiments

Many concerns are raised over inflicting pain and sufferings to animals including sacrifice of animals. These issues are widely debated among various sections of society and in between two extreme views from total banning of animal experiments by animal welfare groups to there is no need of any control or regulations on animal experiments by some researchers, the issue of rational and humane use of experimental animals is most accepted view. It takes care of concerns of both extreme groups There should not be any second thought in mind to minimize pain, sufferings and sacrifices of animal without very sound cause of gaining more valuable outcome may it be in terms of learning or getting answers for hypotheses pertaining to biological sciences.

Two British scientists, Bill Russell and Rex Burch introduced the "3Rs" as framework for considering the humane use of animals. (Russell W. M. S. and Burch R. L. (1959) The principles of humane experimental technique Special Edition, Universities Federation for Animal Welfare, Potters Bar, England). These are- Replace, Reduce and Refine.

REPLACE

Replacement means the substitution for conscious living higher animals of insentient material i.e. replace animal experiments where possible with alternatives. Alternatives which replace animal models can be classified into the following broad general categories: Use of Computer Simulation, Use of Nonliving Systems, and Use of Living Systems.

Use of Computer Simulations: There is controversy due to the claims made for computer simulation as a means of virtually replacing the use of living animals. In simulations, biological phenomenons are to be adapted to a computer model and the basic processes must be expressed in a mathematical formula. After development of formula, an enormous number of variables can be introduced and processed to obtain virtual responses. The success of simulations therefore greatly depends upon the generation of a program using accurate mathematical formula. The more accurate the formula, the more successful is the program. The advantages are- it minimizes use of animals, helps in learning in better way as the simulations are prepared considering ideal situations with minimum or almost no error in experimentation, repeatability of experiments. Disadvantages are- At any time it can not create actual situation of conduction of experiments, it does not allow to learn techniques and skills that can be obtained in normal experimentations, it does not allow to learn from mistakes / errors / changes in conditions during the experiment. A good mix of use of simulations and actual experimentations can help enormously.   The details about some of the available softwares and their usage are given in next chapter.

Use of Nonliving Systems

(a) *Chemical Techniques:* The most widely used nonliving model system involves the use of modern chemical techniques. This is particularly true of the analytical techniques which can be used to identify substances and to determine their concentration or potency. Many Bioassays are now replaced by chemical assays involving modern instrumental techniques thereby saving thousands of animals. Immunochemical techniques use the binding capacity of highly specific antibodies to seek out minute quantities of antigen. A classical example of this technique can be demonstrated by the currently used techniques for identifying bacterial toxins. Toxin identification previously required the injection of as many as several hundred mice with supernatant from cultures of suspected contaminating bacteria.

These new antibody techniques not only save animals but also speed up confirmation of a tentative diagnosis. By adding a colour marker to the Enzyme Linked Immunosorbent Assay system (ELISA), the whole process becomes a commercially available test kit such as those used in home pregnancy detection. A test that previously required the use of a rabbit now can be performed using an over-the-counter test kit. There are a variety of chemical techniques that can be used to determine the presence of a particular chemical reaction or the presence of an enzyme necessary for a specific reaction. At the most basic level, the identification of a particular chemical structure in a compound can provide a great deal of insight into the potential reactivity and thus the resulting toxicity of a given substance.

(b) *Physical and/or Mechanical Systems*: The use of physical and/or mechanical systems to replace living animals of even the highest order has application in teaching specific skills and/or reactions to a well defined set of predetermined circumstances. The use of computer-linked mannequins in teaching basic principles of medicine and applied techniques can be best illustrated by the mannequins used to train people in cardiopulmonary resuscitation.

Use of Living Systems

(a) *In Vitro Techniques:* The most commonly recognized nonanimal living systems are those which fall into the broad category of in vitro methods such as organ, tissue and cell culture. The most commonly used of the in vitro methods are cell culture techniques for monoclonal antibody production, virus vaccine production, vaccine potency testing, screening for the cytopathic effects of various compounds and studying the function and make up of cell membranes. The potential uses of in vitro techniques are almost limitless and will continue to expand as more is learned about the various organs and their component tissues and cells, and as the technology of maintaining in vitro environments improves. Recently due to ban on frog many universities introduced rat experiments. Although it has led to use of higher phylogenetic animals, it has reduced the number of animals as from one rat several pieces of tissue like ileum can be obtained sufficing almost batch of 20-30 students. In addition many other tissues can be simultaneously studied once the animal is sacrificed.

Many academicians have started using tissues from animals/ birds which are killed for meat. e.g. Chicken, goat etc. Chick ileum, goat trachea like tissues are widely used tissues obtained from the butcher's shop (Details to be added in Section for in-vitro preparations in Part –II of the book series). This not only minimizes the animal sacrifice but also helps in reducing difficulties related to regulatory aspects.

(b) *Invertebrate Animals:* Invertebrates are another type of living system which can be used to replace the more commonly used laboratory animals. Over 90 percent of the animal species thus far identified are invertebrates. An invertebrate which has long been used in biomedical research is the fruit fly, *Drosophila melanogaster* -- a classic model for the study of genetics. This species also can be used for detecting mutagenicity, teratogenicity and reproductive toxicity. The marine invertebrates represent different species which have not been widely investigated. However in neurobiology a number of different marine species have been well characterized and used to study the physiology of the nervous system.

(c) *Micro-Organisms:* The micro-organisms represent a third system which has been used to replace traditional animal models. The Ames mutagenicity/carcinogenicity test uses <u>Salmonella</u> <u>typhimurium</u> cultures to screen compounds that formerly required the use of animals. Such systems allow for an almost limitless number of compounds to be tested which can create an interesting dilemma. Alternative techniques can replace the number of animals at a given step in the screening process.

(d) *Plants:*   Plants can offer another alternative living system which may be used to replace animals in studies of basic molecular mechanisms. There is very little morphological and functional difference between the organelles isolated from plants and those isolated from animals. The rigid cell wall of plants, however limits their applicability for use as undisrupted cells.

REDUCE

It means reduction in the numbers of animals used to obtain information of given amount and precision. i. e reduce the number of experiments, and the number of animals in each experiment, to an absolute minimum. In discussing the ways to reduce the numbers of animals used, the definition of an animal and the principle of moving down the phylogentic scale must also be kept in mind. The four broad categories for reducing the number of animals used are: Animal Sharing, Improved Statistical Design, Phylogenetic Reduction, and Better Quality Animals

(a) *Experimental Design:* It can be understood from the forthcoming chapters like computer Assisted Learning and Use of Computers for data analyses about use of statistical tools like power calculations in experimental design. The availability of low cost statistical packages for almost every computer in the market permits more and more investigators access to sophisticated ways of data management and analyses. This accessibility makes possible the use of design criteria and complicated statistical analysis which heretofore have been largely confined to institutions with large statistical support units. With this ability at their finger tips, investigators should be able to maximize the analysis of the data generated from each animal used, thus reducing the total numbers of animals necessary for a particular set of data. Improper design of experimental protocols and/or the failure to use appropriate statistical methods can result in the usage of an inappropriate number of experimental animals. A variety of design strategies are available which can reduce the number of animals needed in a given study. Experimental protocols which utilize serial sacrifice, group sequential testing and crossover designs can significantly reduce the numbers of animals required. In the next chapter topic on Experimental Designs in MICROLAB software explains the importance of power calculation in experimental design in deciding optimum number of animals to be used in experiment.

(b) *Sharing:* Sharing of animals can significantly reduce the number of animals used within a given institution. Sharing can be as simple as allowing someone to practice a surgical approach on an animal that has been, or is to be euthanatized for other purposes, or providing organs or tissues at the time of necropsy. In case studies in the given institute involve the need to perform a sham operation, the administration of compounds by identical routes, the use of standard control diets or the need to condition animals to a particular environment, control animals could be shared within the institution. This can be achieved by regulating body like IEAC to suggest the reduction of animals by sharing whenever it can be feasible.

(c) *Better Quality Animals:* The best quality animal in terms of health status should be used to reduce the possibility that animals will be lost or data compromised by the intrusion of a concurrent disease condition is minimized, if not eliminated. Choosing the best quality animals, in terms of genetic status, will virtually insure the consistency of animals from study to study. This will automatically reduce variations in the results leading to more statistically valid results at the cost of smaller group size. The role of the investigator and staff in assuring the integrity of an animal colony is therefore highly expected. A veterinarian should be consulted to ensure that the best animals that can be effectively maintained in the institution are used during the studies.

(d) *Phylogenetic Reduction:* Use of species from lower biological rank (Phylum forming smaller animal) instead of higher rank is phylogenetic reduction. e. g. using mice instead of rat or using rat instead of rabbits.

REFINEMENT

Experiments that have to be carried out should be refined in such a way that the animals undergo the minimum of discomfort (preferably none at all) and such that the scientific quality is as high as possible. Thus, Refinement means any decrease in the incidence or severity of inhumane procedures applied or application of techniques which can reduce the pain and distress produced in experimental animal. It can be classified into the following broad categories: Decreased Invasiveness, Improved Instrumentation, Improved Control of Pain and Improved Control of Techniques

(a) **Reduction in Invasiveness:** Most of the new diagnostic and therapeutic techniques used in human medicine are aimed at minimising degree of invasiveness e. g. laparoscopic Operations with minimal surgery. Similar techniques can be adopted for use in animals. A sophisticated example could be the use of Magnetic Resonance Imaging for results that formerly required euthanasia of multiple animals along a time curve to obtain assay tissue. Today one animal can provide all the information along a given curve. A less dramatic example is the vascular canula which permits repeated samples or injections in a single animal instead of using several animals. They represent an alternative technique and also help in producing much more consistent and reproducible data.

(b) **Improved Instrumentation**

   (i) *Improved Control of Pain:* While submitting Part-B and protocol to IAEC for approval experimenter has to state that the principal investigator considered alternatives to any procedure likely to produce pain or distress in an experimental animal and plans for the use of agents like- tranquilizers, analgesics and anaesthetics to minimize it unless and until the experimental design does not allow to do so.

   (ii) *Monitoring Animals:* Due to availability of micro and nanoelectronics, fibre optics and laser instrumentation several opportunities for refining techniques used in animal experimentation are available. Improved instrumentation can minimize animal distress by reducing the level of restraint and/or manipulation necessary to obtain biological samples. Included in this category is the use of catheters, wireless transmission system from the implants in animal body emitting signals related to changes in a variety of species allowing continuous access to/ recording changes from the various organ systems, while permitting the animal virtually unrestricted movement within its primary enclosure. The advantages of these systems are numerous like getting real time changes, minimizing a variety of nonexperimental variables associated with prolonged restraint and exclude effects of anaesthesia giving better picture.

   (iii) *Improved Control of Techniques:* The experimenter has to get proficient in various techniques as described in earlier chapter (Chapter-4). It becomes easier to perform a variety of routine procedures with minimal or no pain or distress to the animals involved. Animals are creatures of habit and when proper handling is part of their regular routine, the degree of distress caused by the procedures is minimized which also leads to producing better results as there will be little or no experimental stress. Animals can be trained or conditioned to accept a variety of procedures which if suddenly forced upon them can be distressful. Almost every animal commonly used in the laboratory responds positively to a little tender loving care. To develop the proper techniques and gain confidence in their use requires training by someone with appropriate experience. This can be the veterinarian, a member of the animal care staff or a fellow investigator. Whoever it may be should be sought out before a new species or technique is incorporated into the study. This will reduce the potential distress to all animals involved in the study.

(iv) *Analyzing Samples:* Once obtained, samples can be analyzed in very small volumes for a multitude of parameters. Examples of this can be found in the commercially available diagnostic laboratory equipment which requires only microliter blood samples to perform a variety of diagnostic tests. The use of smaller sample sizes permits the use of smaller animal species and prevents the need to euthanatize many of these species to obtain the necessary volume of blood. It is now possible to obtain serial blood samples from small laboratory rodents which reduce the number of animals necessary to obtain data over the length of the study.

4th R- Many Views

In addition to the 3 R's of Russell and Burch, a fourth R has recently been introduced to the scientific community. The fourth R overlaps some of the refinement techniques. Ronald Banks proposed the 4th R of research as being **Responsibility**. He states, "Responsibility towards research animals focuses new facility design and facility renovation toward accommodation of social interaction and behavioral interplay performing approved experimentation in a manner as distress free as possible, with analgesics or anesthetics used when necessary, of sufficient efficacy and dosage to ameliorate pain and distress." We also share a responsibility to educate the public and show them that we do care about the welfare of the animals. Other Scientists believe that it is **Rehabilitation**- Recently, CPCSEA has made it a national policy that personnel using experimental animals have a moral responsibility towards these animals after their use and most importantly brought forward the concept of the fourth R, "rehabilitation" of used laboratory animals. Costs of aftercare/rehabilitation of animals post experimentation are to be a part of research costs and should be scaled in positive correlation with the level of sentience of the animals. Some think that **Retiring** unwanted (unused or used but not sacrificed) experimental animals to sanctuaries can be the 4th R.

Websites promoting the 3Rs

There are many agencies which either voluntarily, with support from various philanthropic organizations; donors or animals care groups have developed various resources that will promote the principles of 3Rs. Some of these are enlisted below-

1. The National Centre for Replacement, Refinement and Reduction (www.nc3rs.org.uk)

2. Altweb, the Alternatives to Animal Testing Web Site, was created to serve as a gateway to alternatives news, information, and resources on the Internet and beyond (altweb.jhsph.edu).

   The Johns Hopkins Centre for Alternatives to Animal Testing (CAAT) has worked with scientists since 1981 to find new methods to replace the use of laboratory animals in experiments, reduce the number of animals tested, and refine necessary tests to eliminate pain and distress. (caat.jhsph.edu)

3. FRAME (Fund for the Replacement of Animals in Medical Experiments) (www.frame.org.uk). A guide to searching for alternatives is available on the FRAME web site

4. The Dr. Hadwen Trust "... opens the doors to its Science Room website at http://www.scienceroom.org'/

   The Norwegian Reference Centre for Laboratory Animal Science and Alternatives (Laboratory Animal Unit, Norwegian School of Veterinary Science) has maintained a website featuring the NORINA database (www.norinadatabase.org). NORINA is an English language database and contains information on nearly 4,000 audiovisual aids and other material that can be used as alternatives or supplements to animal use in teaching and training. The website also includes TextBase, a database with information on 1100 textbooks of relevance to the three R's. The site includes information on guidelines for animal research, the care and use of fish, and links to databases with the 3 R's.

5. InterNICHE-InterNICHE (**www.interniche.org**) is an international network for humane education. It aims for a high quality, fully humane education in biological science, veterinary and human medicine. It supports progressive science teaching and the

replacement of animal experiments by working with teachers to introduce alternatives, and with students to support freedom of conscience. The types of alternatives offered by InterNICHE include: Models and simulators, Film and video, Multimedia computer simulation

6. The Australian Code of practice for the care and use of animals: NHMRC Australian Code of Practice for the Care and Use of Animals for Scientific Purposes.

Alternative Methodologies in Education and Training (Collective approach using 3 R's)

To summarize, alternative techniques refer to those which can be used in addition to the more traditional animal models. These techniques can focus on specific biological functions and in many cases reduce the numbers of animals used. Therefore these methods are an adjunct to the more commonly used animal models. For others the term **alternative** refers to those techniques which can entirely replace the use of animals.

The working definition of alternative techniques thus evolves to "those techniques which replace the actual use of animals, reduce the numbers used, and/or refine the techniques to minimize the potential for the animal to experience pain or distress."

Here alternative techniques included non-recovery techniques in anesthetized animals, as well as tissue culture, as replacement methods. Reduction included statistical techniques which were designed to reduce the actual numbers needed in the study. The use of better animals was also encouraged as a means of reducing actual numbers used. Refinement referred to techniques that reduced the potential for pain and distress. In recent years there has been considerable evolution of alternatives in education and training and the realization that animal use is not essential to many components of the teaching of science, of veterinary medicine and of medicine. The emerging range of alternatives is impressive and few examples of this range are detailed below.

Models and simulators

These range from inexpensive models and surgical training devices, right up to costly computerised mannequins. Basic models can contribute to the study of anatomy or facilitate the learning of good animal handling without animal stress and student anxiety. The diversity of surgical training devices available include models of skin, internal organs and limbs which can provide opportunities for students to master basic skills such as eye-hand co-ordination, the use of instruments, and techniques such as suturing. Waste organ training devices allow for the use of real tissue in the process. More complex products include mannequins used to train IV skills, intubation and catheterisation of animals. Computerised mannequins add another level of complexity and support to the effective training of students.

Film and Video

Film and video can give good background and provide a quality audio-visual alternative. Videos of professionally performed experiments can often impart much more information to students than experiments performed by the students themselves and can be used to train those students who need such skills in their careers before they perform such experiments. Few very good examples can be perused in next chapter giving information about CALs showing various visuals about Dog BP experiment and effects of drugs on behaviour of animals etc.

Multimedia computer simulation

There are many computer simulation programmes available to teach various experiments there by minimizing the use of animals. Some programmes include virtual laboratories with options for working through different experiments, and others can be customised by teachers to adapt them to the location and to specific teaching objectives. Wherever possible, however, computer simulation should be used in tandem with experience of living people or non-human animals so that technology is kept as a powerful tool, not an alternative to reality. The details about such few freely available softwares are given in next chapter.

The InterNICHE Alternatives Loan System

The InterNICHE Alternatives Loan System is an evolving library of multimedia CD-ROMs, videos, models and mannequins. It covers fields such as anatomy, physiology and surgery. Teachers and students from anywhere in the world can borrow items from the Loan System to trial them. This gives user the opportunity to familiarise themselves with some of the best products available. All items in the Loan System have been chosen with reference to meeting teaching objectives for practical classes to shift the emphasis away from the invasive animal lab towards alternative approaches.

The NORINA Database

Alternatives to the Use of Animals for Toxicity Testing

Increasingly validated alternatives to sentient animals are being used in the field of toxicity testing. With reference to the Australian veterinary situation the Australian Pesticides and Veterinary Medicines Authority websites states that experiments involving animals should be conducted with the minimum number of animals necessary to allow valid conclusions to be drawn.

Applicants are encouraged to submit data obtained in *in-vitro* assay systems, or from alternative methods which use fewer animals, as a means of facilitating validation of alternate methodologies and reducing the number of animals used in toxicity testing.

Before commencement of toxicology studies, and with regard to possible alternatives to animals reference to relevant data bases should be made. There are a number of websites that may be similarly referred to. In 1997 the John Hopkins Centre for Alternatives to Animal Testing (CAAT) launched Altweb, the Alternatives to Animal Testing Web Site (http:altweb.jhsp.edu). Altweb was created to serve as a central reference point or gateway to alternatives information, resources and news. It is international in scope and freely available.

Alternatives in toxicology research for humans

The European Medicines Agency (EMEA, http://www.emea.eu.int/) is a decentralised body of the European Union responsible for the protection and promotion of public and animal health, through the evaluation and supervision of medicines for human and veterinary use. The Committee for Medicinal Products for Human Use (CHMP) has prepared a document reviewing the use of alternative, genetically modified animal models for carcinogenicity testing

(http://www.emea.eu.int/pdfs/human/swp/259202en.pdf). The European Centre for the Validation of Alternative Methods (ECVAM, http://ecvam.jrc.it/index.htm) is responsible for coordinating the validation of alternative test methods in the EU. Its website can be searched for validated alternative tests and information on alternatives for scientific and regulatory purposes.

A comparable organisation in the USA is the Interagency Coordinating Committee on the Validation of Alternative Methods (ICCVAM) (http://iccvam.niehs.nih.gov/). The National Institute of Environmental Health Sciences (NIEHS) established the ICCVAM to develop and validate new test methods, and to establish criteria and processes for the validation and regulatory acceptance of toxicological testing methods. The National Toxicology Program (NTP, http://ntp.niehs.nih.gov/ntpweb/index.cfm?objectid=7182FF48-BDB7-CEBA-F8980E5DD01A1E2D) Interagency Centre for the Evaluation of Alternative Toxicological Methods (NICEATM) was established to provide operational support for ICCVAM. The ICCVAM web site can be searched for alternative test methods and information. Replacement alternatives in toxicology have evolved rapidly in recent times. The processes of method development, pre-validation and validation have reached a level of international consensus. When it comes to replacement methods, biomedical research presents different challenges and opportunities and investigations are more open ended.

The Netherlands Centre for Alternatives to Animal Use identifies two groups of replacement alternatives: relative and absolute replacement models. Relative replacement alternatives still require an animal for the donation of organs tissues or cells. Absolute replacement models have no vertebrate animal involvement.

There are several non-animal methods currently used in biomedical research:

(a) prior information (databases)

(b) computer modelling

(c) bio kinetic modelling

(d) the use of new molecular biology technologies (genomics, proteomics, metabonomics)

(e) in vitro models (cells, tissues, organs)

(f) human studies

It is also possible to replace technologies used in animals by in-vitro alternatives. As an example of replacement of a technology that can provide pain and distress in animals, the ascites fluid method of monoclonal antibody production is no longer acceptable, and must be replaced by in-vitro methods, except in rare cases where in vitro methods are shown to be unsuitable.

8

Computer Assisted Learning

The previous chapter dealt with humane approach for using animals for experiments by adopting 4 R's. The opportunities associated with the development of computer software in contributing to effective life science education have grown exponentially within the last few years. From virtual dissections that students can perform on-screen, to full virtual reality simulations of clinical technique with 3-D and tactile facilities, the possibilities are limited only by technical and imaginative boundaries. Computer-assisted learning can also offer much greater depth and breadth to the learning experience. Accordingly many efforts are made to use computer aided or assisted learning (CAL) enabling students and teachers to minimize use of animals for learning. Many scientist simulated variety of animal experiments which not only help in understanding the experiment in better way but also give chance to perform again and again with different modes. Students can also work at their own pace, repeat parts of the exercise and use the support material until they are confident with knowledge and technique, and be as self-directed as the structure of the course allows. The innovative nature of new technological developments can be exciting, which adds to the learning experience for students and is an important part of their informal training for professions where IT and computer skills will continue to play a major role. Although no software can replace actual experience obtained during performing experiment, it definitely has edge over going for direct animal experiment when ever simulations for such experiments are available. Teacher can demonstrate experiments using CAL and after building confidence actual experiments can be performed. Previous demonstration using such softwares can minimize fear of animal handling, stigma of handling / sacrificing animal and time to learn the technique. Most of the undergraduate students face difficulty during Pharmacology experiments and such software/s can help to remove their inhibitions. In some places animal experiments could be conducted and if at all conducted, they are done with great difficulties because of regulatory aspects like-CPCSEA permission; approval by IAEC; availability of animals in addition to availability of facility including trained staff. Taking cognisance of above cited difficulties and benefits many universities have prescribed some experiments based on simulation in addition to routine experiments. The Pharmacy Council of India also recommended use of simulation for the same purpose.

Many such softwares are available either Free or Paid. In this book efforts are made to introduce some of the freely available softwares with respect to their availability, mode of usage and applications. In India great efforts are made by Dr.R.Raveendran, (Former Editor, IJP and Professor, Department of Pharmacology, JIPMER, Pondicherry) by preparing many types of software, distributing his and some other softwares freely either along with issues of Indian Journal of Pharmacology (during his tenure as chief- editor of journal) or by making it available for free downloads from INdphar website http://www.ampiweb.org/indphar/sware.htm. Most important aspects of these softwares are they provide experiments of different animals like frog, rat, guinea pig, rabbit, cat and even dog in addition to facts that these are easy to use, reviewed for their appropriateness and if needed examinations can also be conducted (using either paid versions or versions distributed freely with journal).

How to use-The text below screen shots/ figures of different software describes the steps to be followed at the time of use. For the ease alphabets and numbers are put on the figures and in same order the text is described below the figure.

I. **ExPharm** is a CAL (Computer Assisted Learning) package containing four programs which simulate some of the animal experiments in Pharmacology. These programs can be used to demonstrate drug actions on different animal systems. The package is user friendly, highly interactive and full of animated sequences which make simulation appear realistic. It will be useful especially in places where the use of animals for teaching is banned or restricted due to various reasons.

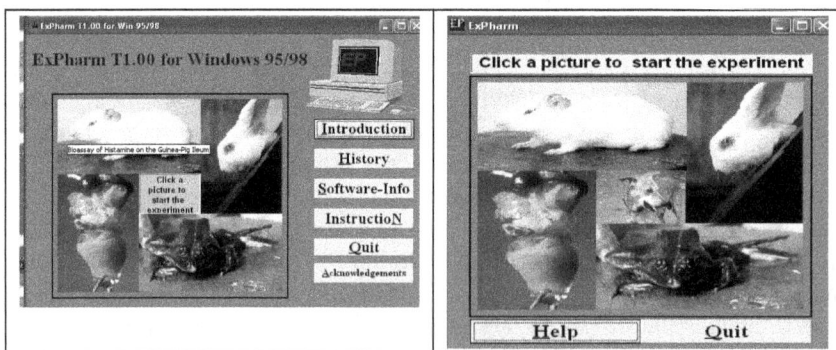

ExPharm T1 version consists of four programs:

1. Effects of drugs on the rabbit eye
2. Effects of drugs on the frog heart

3. Effects of drugs on the frog oesophagus

4. Bioassay of histamine using guinea pig ileum

The T2 version is having dog BP as additional programme

One should click on image of desired experiment to start the programme.

For other details one can click other links like Introduction, history, Software info, Introduction etc and Quit if wish to exit the programme.

There are two versions, T1.00 for Windows 95/98. In which Examination mode is disabled and one can run the experiments in Tutorial mode only. The other one is E version. The package is available on CDs (from Dr.R.Raveendran) or can be downloaded from the website http://www.ampiweb.org/indphar/sware.htm. The pharmacologists / colleges receiving Indian Journal of Pharmacology must be having it as it was offered free with Indian Journal of Pharmacology Issue one in **Issue 6 Volume 35 December 2003 and** second time December 2006 issue. Recently T2 version is launched which can be downloaded from the IndPhar website. This includes Dog BP (One need not to run dog BP software separately unless the person wants to see the VDOs) and help files are PDF files

I. 1.   Rabbit- Effects of drugs on the Rabbit eye

The software simulates the actions drugs such as physostigmine, atropine, ephedrine, epinephrine and lignocaine on pupil size, corneal and pupillary reflexes and intraocular tension. The user can instil the drugs on the eye and observe their effects which can be compared with saline effect. He/she can test the reflexes using a torch and a cotton wool provided. The intraocular tension is indicated. The readings can be noted and a table of observations can be made using the model table provided. Examination mode has two modules. One deals with identification of unknown drugs based on their effects. The other involves designing an experiment to find out whether the unknown drug produces any effect on the pupil. This mode is available in version E1.00 only.

Basis behind study

The Iris is composed of two types of muscle fibres, the circular and the radial. The circular fibres are supplied by parasympathetic nerve fibres and the radial ones are innervated by sympathetic nerve fibres. The stimulation of sympathetic and parasympathetic nerves produces mydriasis and miosis respectively and their paralysis produces opposite effects. Further being a delicate and important organ, very strong reflexes are observed if some object comes close to eye. Agents like anaesthetics minimises this reflexes.

Drugs which simulate the effects of autonomic nervous system can produce the above mentioned effects. This experiment uses a few such drugs on the rabbit eye like - 1. Normal saline, 2. Physostigmine (0.5%), 3. Atropine sulphate (1.0%), 4. Ephedrine (0.5%), 5. Adrenaline hydrochloride (0.1%), 6. Lignocaine hydrochloride (1.0%)

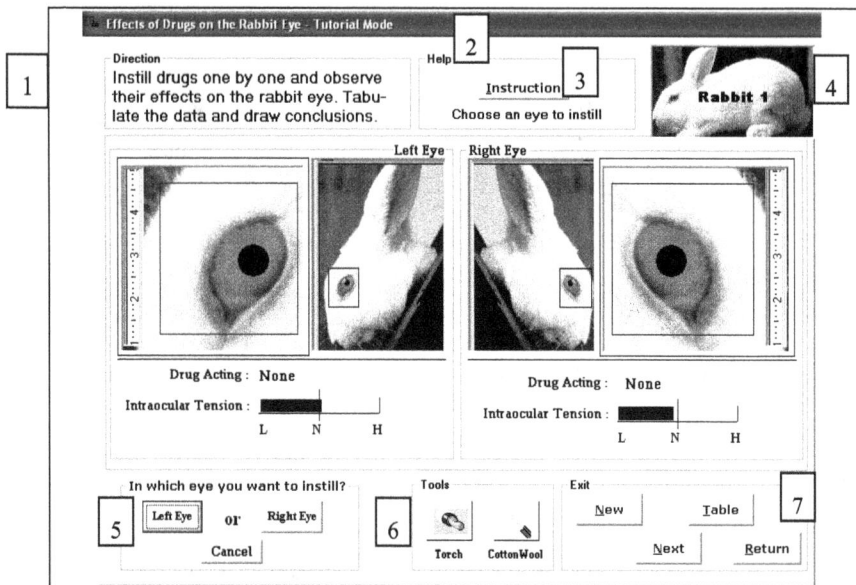

1. Direction- It directs about next steps to be followed.
2. Help- Provides Help
3. Introduction- Introduces the experiment concept
4. Displays Rabbit Number which is used for experiment at the given instance.

   In 4 boxes images of left eye and right eye displayed with their enlarged images. The enlarged images are also equipped with scale to measure the pupil size.

   Below each eye the information about which drug is acting is displayed.

   The horizontal bar displays changes in intraocular pressure (IOP) from Low to High Below are several buttons for various functions.
5. Gives choice to select eye, although both eyes can be used better to use one eye at a time to observe the difference.
6. Offers tools to check activities. Torch to note changes in pupil size and cotton wool to measure reflexes.
7. Exit box-includes the following buttons-New - to change the rabbit, Table - to display model table, Next - to end the experiment, Return-to abort and be back to main menu.

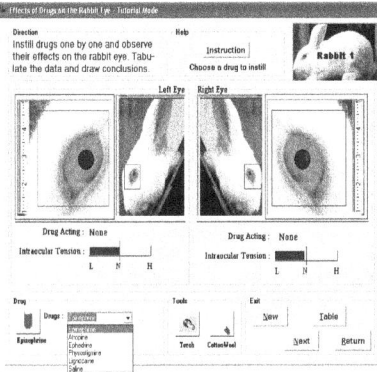

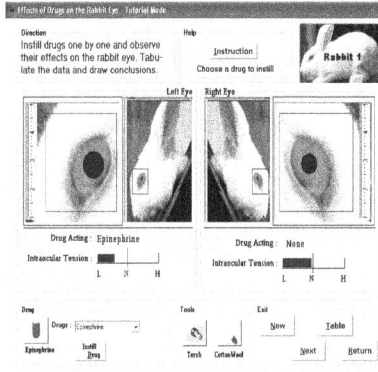

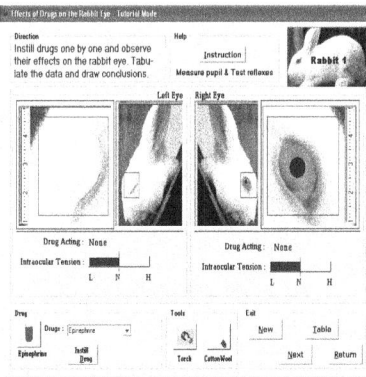

Note the changes-After selecting animal (see 5 in Fig. 6.1) the Drug button is visible which gives various options. See the example above selecting epinephrine as drug instilled in left eye showing reduction in IOP. Click torch or cotton wool and take it to eyes to see reflex along with effect of drugs on reflexes. Important suggestions-Use saline control for all drugs, Measurements must be recorded before and after adding saline or drugs, Use only one drug on a rabbit. Use fresh rabbits to test drugs, Use the scale provided to measure the pupil size (Each division is1 mm).

I. 2. ExPharm-Heart ver T1.01 Effects of Drugs on the Isolated Heart of Frog

The software simulates the actions of drugs such as epinephrine (adrenaline), norepinephrine (noradrenaline), isoprenaline, propranolol, acetylcholine, atropine, calcium chloride and potassium chloride on heart rate, tone and force (amplitude) of contraction using isolated frog heart. The user can inject drugs and observe their effect(s) which can be compared with that of Ringer. The readings can be noted and a table of observations can be made using the model table provided.

Basis behind study

Many drugs act on the heart. Adrenergic and cholinergic drugs produce opposite effects on it through respective receptors. Some drugs act directly on the heart. This experiment demonstrates the effects of following drugs (agonists, antagonists, calcium and potassium) on the isolated heart of frog.

SOLUTIONS and DRUGS

	Dose (mcg)	Concentration (mcg/ml)
1. Frog-Ringer	-	-
2. Epinephrine (Adrenaline)	2	10
3. Norepinephrine (Noradrenaline)	2	10
4. Isoprenaline	2	10
5. Propranolol	200	1 mg/ml
6. Acetylcholine	2	10
7. Atropine sulphate	20	100
8. Calcium Chloride	2000	10 mg/ml
9. Potassium Chloride	2000	10 mg/ml

Volume of above solutions to be injected = 0.2 ml   mcg   =   micrograms (mg)

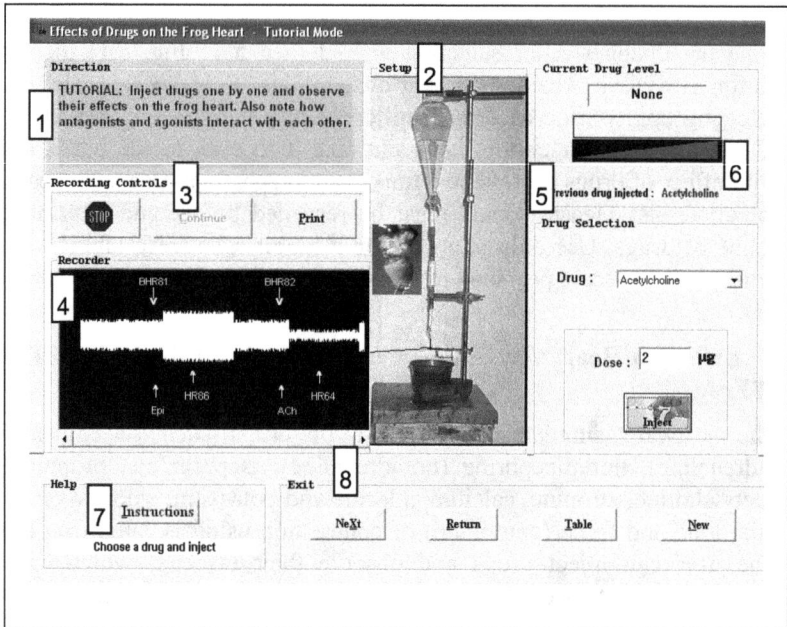

1. Direction Box - displays directions for experiments.
2. Set up Box -displays set up of isolated heart preparation and equipment.
3. Recorder control- displays drum controls such as Stop, Continue and Print.
4. Recorder Box- displays drum on which the recordings are seen.
5. Drug selection Box- displays drugs list and the drug and the dose selected. The user can choose the drug and inject also.
6. Drug level Box- displays the level of current drug injected. Before the drug gets out of the heart, another drug can be injected and interaction between two drugs can be demonstrated. The last drug injected is also displayed.
7. Help box-displays instruction button which on clicking can show this page.
8. Exit box - displays controls such as Next, Return, Table and New.

   Next - displays questions. Return - returns user to menu page

   Table - displays model table. New - starts a new experiment.

Drugs are injected (one by one) into the Ringer piercing the rubber tube and contractions are recorded on the chart. The heart rate (beats/min) is counted and noted on the chart. The event of drug administration is also marked on the chart.

Methodology[1]

Inject drugs one by one. Observe the following before and after drug administration:

   (a) Force of contraction - amplitude (normal, increased or decreased),

   (b) tone (normal, increased or decreased),

   (c) heart rate (beats per minute)

Parameter (a) and (b) are assessed by observing the recording. The amplitude of contractions reflects the force. Shift in the mid point of systolic and diastolic contractions indicate the change in tone.

Precautions

---

[1] Methodology- In this chapter methodology means the steps suggested by the programmer of that software to be followed while using given software. The details are explained with provision of numbers/alphabets on figure and matching it in text.

(a) Wait till contractions appear on the chart before administering drugs.

(b) Give sufficient time for the heart to recover between drug administrations.

(c) Always note the parameter readings before and after giving drugs.

(d) One cannot mix two drugs and inject. The drugs should be given one by one. When a drug is given, its level is displayed. This gives a rough indication of when the action of the drug ends. If the next drug is given before the action of current drug is over, the interaction can be seen. Please note: The interactions between agonists and antagonists can be observed. However the potentiation between adrenergic drugs may not be seen clearly.

(e) The doses are fixed. Do not give a drug repeatedly in order to increase the dose.

I. 3.   ExPharm-Oesophagus ver T1.00 Effect of drugs on the ciliary motility of frog oesophagus

The software simulates effect of drugs on ciliary motility of the frog oesophagus and the action of drugs such as acetylcholine, physostigmine and atropine on it. The user can instill the drugs on the dissected oesophagus and observe their effect on ciliary motility by measuring the movement of poppy seeds placed at the cephalic end of oesophagus. The time taken for the seed to move a fixed distance on the oesophagus can be noted with the help of a clock / stop watch. The time taken by the seeds measured after application of frog-Ringer (control) and drug (test) can be compared.

Basis behind study

Frog oesophagus contains cilia. Ciliary motility depends on action of acetylcholine in mucous membrane. ACh causes contraction of cilia leading to increased movements. Cholinergic drugs produce similar effect while anticholinergics paralyze cilia and decrease their movements. This experiment deals with a few such drugs to demonstrate their effect using given drugs & solutions- 1. Acetylcholine (10%), 2. Physostigmine (10%), 3. Atropine (0.1%) and 4. Frog Ringer

Set up- It simulates experiment on a frog, which is pithed and lower jaw is removed. The oesophagus is slit open from buccal cavity to the stomach and everted to fix it on a wooden board with pins. Blood is wiped away by a cotton swab dipped in frog Ringer solution. The surface is moistened with frog Ringer. A poppy seed is placed at the cephalic end and its movements and time taken to travel a fixed distance on the oesophagus are observed.

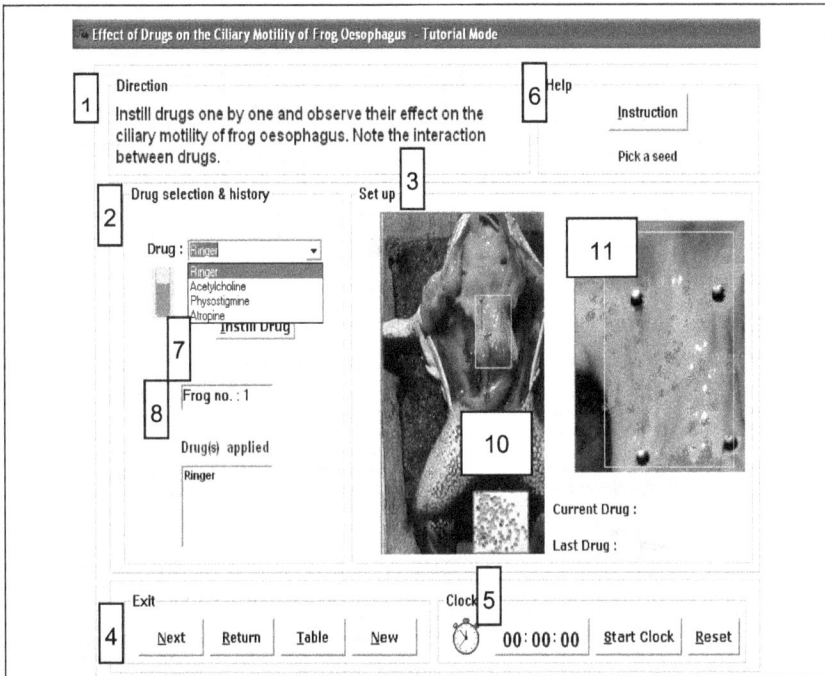

10. Pick & place a poppy Seed: Click on pick a seed (below instruction tab).Take the cursor to poppy seeds and click the mouse. A seed will be picked up. Without releasing the mouse button, drag the seed on to oesophagus and place it at an appropriate area (cephalic end) on the oesophagus. The seed will be seen moving on the enlarged image of the oesophagus.

1. Direction Box-displays direction to do the experiment.

2. Drug selection & history Box- helps to choose the drug and instill it on the oesophagus. Indicates the frog (preparation) number currently in use. Drug history (drug application) is displayed.

3. Set up Box-displays the animal system dissected and set up for experimentation. Shows poppy seeds also. A portion of the oesophagus is enlarged and displayed to observe the movement of poppy seed clearly.

4. Exit Box-includes the following buttons. Click *New-* to start a new experiment. *Table* - to display model table. *Next* - to end the experiment. *Return* - to abort and be back to main menu.

5. Clock Box-Shows the clock that can be started/stopped by clicking 'Start Clock' button .Clock can be reset to 00:00:00 by clicking 'Reset' button.

6. Help Box-Click 'Help' to view this page. Short instructions / guidance will also appear on the box. Ignore them when they are not appropriate.

7. Instill drug: - Choose a drug and click instill button. One will see a dropper instilling the drug on the oesophagus. Frog-Ringer will be automatically instilled at the start of the experiment to prevent drying up of the tissue.

8. Displays the Frog used- First, second etc

9. Box giving information about drugs applied on oesophagus.

10. Pick & place a poppy seed- See below figure

11. Enlarged view of oesophagus and pins. The observations of descend of poppy seeds from cephalic pins to distal pins to be made using the enlarged view

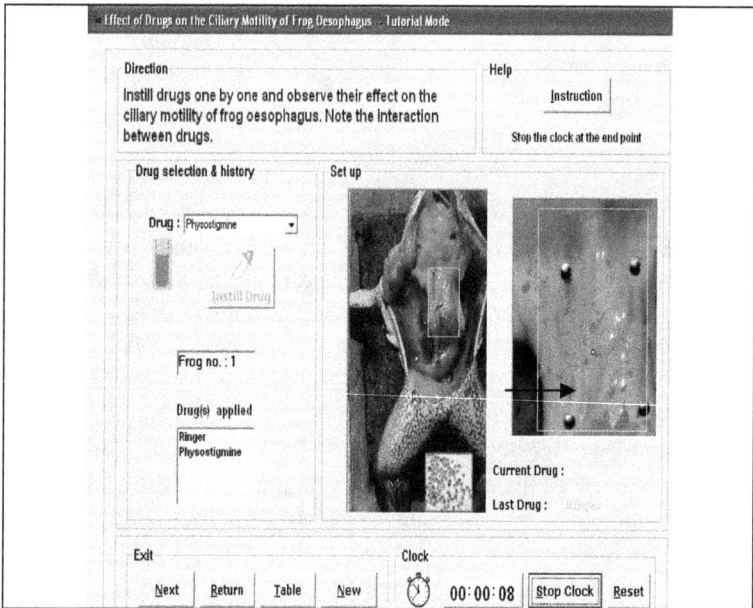

Black arrow indicating poppy seed descending down.

Methodology

1. Determine the distance of seed movement. The starting point and the end point will be pins fixed at the cephalic end and caudal (distal) end respectively.

2. Instill frog-Ringer on the surface of the oesophagus. Place a poppy seed at the cephalic end of oesophagus. The seed starts moving due to ciliary motility. When the seed crosses the starting point (cephalic end pins), start the stop clock. Stop it when the seed reaches the distal pins.
3. Note down the time taken for the seed to travel the distance. Repeat step 2 to get three readings. Calculate the average. This will be control.
4. Instill ACh and take three readings. 5. Repeat step 2 and 3.
6. Instill physostigmine and take three readings. 7. Repeat step 2 and 3.
7. Instill atropine and take three readings.
8. Instill ACh (without using frog-Ringer after step 6) and observe its effect. Compare it with the effect obtained with ACh alone (step 4).

Note:

1. Test each drug including Ringer thrice and calculate average reading for each drug.
2. Readings with Ringer are taken as control and compared with test (drug) readings.
3. Take separate control readings for each drug i.e. Before testing any drug, take readings with Ringer.
4. Use new preparations (frog) for each drug. To observe interactions, drugs should be applied on the same preparation (frog) consecutively without using Ringer in between them.

I. 4.   Bioassay of Histamine on Guinea pig ileum

The details about Bioassay are mentioned in chapter 9. This simulation demonstrates graded dose response and matching assay of histamine on the guinea-pig ileum.

1. Direction box-   displays direction to do the experiment.
2. Help box-shows instructions
3. Recorder box- simulates chart recorder. The curves start appearing from the right margin and move towards left. A scale is provided to measure the height of the curves. Each division represents 0.25 cm.
4. Set up box-shows water bath and organ bath. The tissue is tied to a force transducer which is connected to the chart recorder.
5. Dose selection box- helps to choose the drug (histamine) dose and inject it into the organ bath.
6. Do box   - displays two separate buttons for Printing the graph and starting the MATCHING ASSAY.
7. Exit box-includes the following buttons. Click- New - to start a new experiment. Next - to end the experiment. Return - to abort and be back to main menu.
   - Choose the dose and press inject button. Clicking the buttons + and - will double or halve the dose. The dose can be manually entered by clicking into the dose box.
   - Once the dose response curve is obtained, click the button 'Matching Assay' in Do box. One will be asked to enter the dose of standard curve. Then a panel with the following buttons appears:
     1. Standard 2. Double-Standard 3. Half-Standard 4. Unknown

Clicking buttons 1-3 will inject the respective dose of the standard. No.1 will inject the full dose of the standard selected by the student, no. 2 will double the dose and no. 3 will injects half the dose of standard.

Before pressing unknown button, the dose of unknown in ml has to be selected. This can be done at the Dose selection box. Click the unknown button to inject the selected dose of unknown.
   - After matching, press 'Calculate' button and enter the volume of unknown needed to match. The concentration of histamine in the unknown solution is calculated displayed.
   - After completion, click 'Next'.

Methodology

1. Choose a dose of histamine and inject. Obtain a dose response curve by increasing the dose in geometric progression. The starting dose can be 0.1 mcg. If the tissue is very sensitive start from 0.01 mcg.

   Drug being injected into the organ bath.
2. Once the maximum response is reached, start the matching assay.
3. When one start the matching assay he/she will be given a solution of unknown concentration of histamine. The user will have to choose a standard curve (standard) from his / her dose response curve and enter the amount of histamine (in mcg) which produced the standard curve. The

standard curve is chosen on the basis that the response produced by the curve is about 50% of maximal response (maximal response is one which does NOT increase further with an increase in the dose).

4. Then inject the standard and the unknown alternatively. The unknown is given in ml. The starting dose can be 0.1 ml. Adjust the dose of unknown until it matches with the standard. Matching is achieved by trial and error.

5. Matching can be confirmed by giving 2s or s/2. (double or half the amount of standard) and half or double the dose of unknown that matches the standard. After matching is confirmed, calculate the concentration of histamine in the unknown solution

II. DOG BP

SET UP: A dog is weighed and anaesthetized using intravenous chloralose (100 mg/kg of body weight). It is fixed on a dog table in supine position. Right femoral vein is cannulated with a catheter to inject drugs. Its neck is dissected to expose carotid arteries and vagus nerves. Left common carotid is inserted with an arterial cannula connected to a mercury manometer or to a pressure transducer, which is connected to a polyrite / physiograph. A chart recorder or a kymograph is set up to receive signals from the polyrite/physiograph to produce graphical representation of changes in blood pressure. The left side vagus is cut into central and peripheral ends for applying electrical stimulation later in the experiment. The right common carotid is identified and exposed for later use.

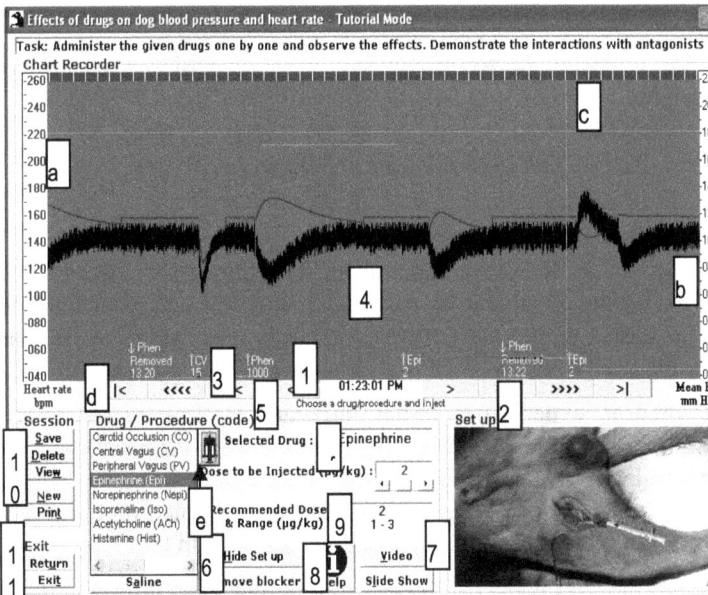

a.   The upper red line indicates heart rate, corresponding to red markings to the right side.

b.   The recording shows change in blood pressure in response to drug/ procedure applied (d), corresponding to black markings to the left side. (c). The movable cursor gives values at selected place. d. The drug / procedure (as mentioned in table) to be selected and administered by pressing injection syringe sign (e) and in given dose/ duration (f)

1.   Direction Box displays directions for experiments.

2.   Set up Box displays pictures of dog preparation set up and equipment.

3.   Recorder control displays drum controls for moving the chart left and right.

4.   Recorder Box displays drum on which the recordings are seen.

5.   Drug selection Box displays drugs list and the drug and the dose selected. The user can choose a drug and inject.
     This box also includes the following buttons:

6.   Hide Set up - the set up can be hidden if the user is not comfortable with the pictures displayed.

7.   Video -run a video Or slide show of dog experiment.

8.   Remove Blocker- the influence of blockers currently acting in the system can be removed. Available in the Tutorial mode only. Slide Show - a series of pictures showing the set up and equipment can be displayed.

9.   Help - displays help pages.

10. Session Box   displays the following controls:
     Save - saves the recording of the current session.
     Delete - deletes the recordings saved on the hard disk during previous sessions.
     View - old recordings saved on the disk can be viewed.
     New - starts a new session of the experiment.
     Print - prints the recording in black & white only.

11. Exit Box -Displays 'Return' and 'Exit':
     Return - takes the user to main menu. This button is replaced by 'Reveal' button in the Examination mode to reveal the nature of the unknown drug. Exit - closes the software. (This is now added in ExPharm T2 version (EPT2) except VDOs/slide shows of the experiment.)

The present experiment which simulates a live anaesthetized dog demonstrates the effects of following drugs on the cardiovascular system. Drugs are injected (one by one) into the femoral vein and BP is recorded on the chart. The heart rate (beats/min) is counted and noted on the chart. Drug administration is also marked which can be observed in the figure above.

Observe the following parameters before and after drug administration: (a) BP (mm of Hg) (b) HR (beats per minute)

Parameters (a) and (b) are assessed by observing the recording. The BP recordings are indicated in black and that of the HR in red. Two scales for measuring BP and HR are provided one at each side of the chart. The one in which the measurements are marked in red indicates HR (beats/min) and the other with black marking indicates BP (mm Hg). Moving the mouse pointer over the chart will display a crosshair that helps to measure the correct BP and HR at given point. The effects can be summarised as follows in Table 8.1.

Nature	Drug name (Dose in mg/kg)	Effect of drug that can be observed after administration as per given instruction
Agonist	Epinephrine Code : Epi Dose : 2, Range : 1 - 3	Adrenaline stimulates the α and β adrenergic receptors. Conventional doses will increase the BP followed by a short fall before reaching the basal level (biphasic response due to α and β receptor responses). To see the β action alone, use a low dose such as 0.1 mg per kg of body weight.
Agonist	Nor-epinephrine Code : Nepi Dose : 3, Range : 2 - 5	Noradrenaline stimulates mainly the α and β1 receptors. The heart rate is generally reduced due to vagal reflex in response to increased BP. Hence if the dog is pretreated with a muscarinic blocker (atropine), norepinephrine will show an increase in the heart rate.
Agonist	Isoprenaline Code : Iso Dose : 3, Range : 2 - 5	Isoproterenol is a potent, non-selective β adrenergic stimulant. It increases the systolic BP (sometimes it remains unchanged) but decreases the diastolic BP. Because the decrease is more pronounced than the increase, the mean arterial pressure typically falls.
Agonist	Acetylcholine Code : Ach Dose : 5, Range : 2 - 10	Intravenous administration of Acetylcholine (ACh) leads to a sharp a fall in BP which returns to basal level quickly. Though ACh generally reduces heart rate, small doses may generally lead to reflex tachycardia. After complete atropinization (this might require a higher dose of atropine), a large dose of ACh (150 - 200 mg/kg) may be tried to demonstrate the 'Nicotinic or Ganglionic' action.
Agonist	Histamine Code : Hist Dose : 3,Range : 2 - 5	Acts on H_1 and H_2 receptors to produce a fall in BP which may be completely blocked when H1 and H2 antagonists are acting concurrently. Either of the antagonists, if given alone will produce only a partial block. Stimulation of H_1 produces a rapid onset short lived decrease in BP whereas H_2 stimulation leads to a fall characterized by slower onset and longer duration.

Contd....

Nature	Drug name (Dose in mg/kg)	Effect of drug that can be observed after administration as per given instruction
Agonist	Ephedrine Code : Ephe Dose : 100, Range : 100 - 200	It acts on both α and β receptors and in addition enhances the release of norepinephrine from sympathetic neurons. It increases the BP and heart rate. Repeated administration within a short time will lead to a gradual decrease in response. This is known as tachyphylaxis. To demonstrate this phenomenon, repeat a conventional dose 4 to 5 times without allowing a large interval between doses.
Antagonist	Phentolamine Code : Phen Dose : 1000	An α blocker drug, reduces BP and also affects the α components of other drugs.
Antagonist	Propranolol Code : Prop Dose : 1000	It is a β blocker which reduces BP and heart rate. It affects the β components of other drugs.
Antagonist	Atropine Code : Atro Dose : 750 Range : 500 - 1000	This drug is a muscarinic cholinergic antagonist. It competitively antagonizes ACh. Atropine in conventional doses may not completely block muscarinic receptors. It may require a higher dose ranging from 1000 to 1500 mg/kg. To demonstrate the nicotinic action of ACh, complete atropinization is a must.
Antagonist	Mepyramine Code : Mep Dose : 5000	Mepyramine is a H_1 blocker. It does not have any action on the CVS but when given alone it blocks partially the fall in BP by histamine.
Antagonist	Cimetidine Code : Cime Dose : 5000	It is a H_2 blocker, which also partially blocks the effect of histamine on BP.
Not known	Unknown Code : Unkn, Dose : 0.1 ml, Range : 0.1 - 0.2 ml	Unknown solution contains one of the drugs listed above. It is randomly chosen by the software and varies each time the user runs the experiment. Unknown solution is given only when the software is run in Examination mode. It contains only one drug.
Neutral Saline	Code : Sal Dose : 1ml Range : 1 - 2 ml	While conducting the live experiment, a small volume of saline is administered following every drug injection, so that the drug remaining in the catheter can be flushed completely into the system.

III.   Microlabs for Pharmacologists

This is again a great gift from Indian Journal of Pharmacology (**Issue 6 Volume 35 December 2003**) along with other softwares. The beauty of the software is that it provides great range of experiments from in-vitro to in-vivo, from mouse to human beings, from simulations to beautiful videos showing effect of variety of drugs and other activities. I believe that it is must for any Pharmacologists to use the software and demonstrate all its modules. Microlabs consists of a series of computer based modules with the primary aim to replace animal use in education by simulating the effects of drugs on isolated tissues (*in vitro)* and on whole animals (*in vivo)*. It allows the user to design experiments and reduce the use of animals by careful planning, to link animal behaviour to pharmacokinetics, to study the effect of drugs and 'unknowns' *in vivo* and *in vitro*, to get information about drugs, and to refine experiments under simulated conditions. **The Author of the software is** Dr.Henk van Wilgenburg, Department of Pharmacology, University of Amsterdam, Amsterdam, and The Netherlands. The total disk space needed for media files is about 570 MB. After installation open the Microlabs directory (**C:\Program Files\Microlab) and click the file microlab.exe to run the software.**

Some of the programs available in the Microlabs package are:

III. 1. Animal behaviour, III. 2. Mouse behaviour, III. 3 Experimental Design, III. 4. Probit Analysis, III. 5. Anaesthesia of the rat, III. 6. Human case studies and pharmacokinetics, III. 7. Guinea pig ileum *in vitro,* III. 8. Phrenic nerve-diaphragm *in vitro*

III. 1. Animal Behaviour

This is a treasure hunt for a Pharmacologist enabling him to watch video clippings of several behavioural patterns that are commonly referred in experimental Pharmacology literature. After opening Microlab as mentioned above, click on first set of simulations after introduction i.e. Animal Behaviour. This will ask permission to Run software symptoms.exe, click yes and it will open second window "SYMPTOMALOGY FOR SUBSTANCES". In this click on initiate which will ask the person to enter Drive name in which Microlab files are installed at the time of installation. Usually it is C drive and after entering C it will give 2 Options Symptoms of lab Animals and Mouse Watch. Clicking the first one brings opens new window SYMPTOMS which having 4 boxes, upper two for showing video clips and lower two for descriptions of above videos. The First box provides videos as per symptoms and provides list of symptoms (peculiar observation) named as- Arched back, Ataxia, Catalepsy, Circling, Control mouse, Control mouse, Dyspnoea, Flat body posture, Forepaws treading, Grooming,

Hypertonia, Hypotonia, Lower lip retraction, Miosis, Mydriasis, Opisthotonus, Piloerection, Ptosis, Rearing, Salivation, Salivation, Spasms, Straub tail, Stereotypies, Tonic convulsion, Tremor, Wet-dog shakes, Writhing syndrome in mouse and in second upper box the videos of effects various drugs like- 5-HT, amphetamine, apomorphine, barbiturate, cannabis, chlorpromazine, clonidine, cocaine, desmethyl imipramine (DMI), diazepam, ether, haloperidol,hexobarbital, morphine, Nicotine, oxotremorine, pentobarbitone, Pentylenetetrazole (leptazole), Picrotoxin, Pilocarpine, Strychnine, thioridazine on various behavioural patterns are given. Below each upper box the information about the activity is described.

The figure given below demonstrates the sample activities- Straub Tail in Symptom box with information in the box given below and Substance (Drug effects) box showing effect of Thioridazine in mice (catalepsy) with information in box given below.

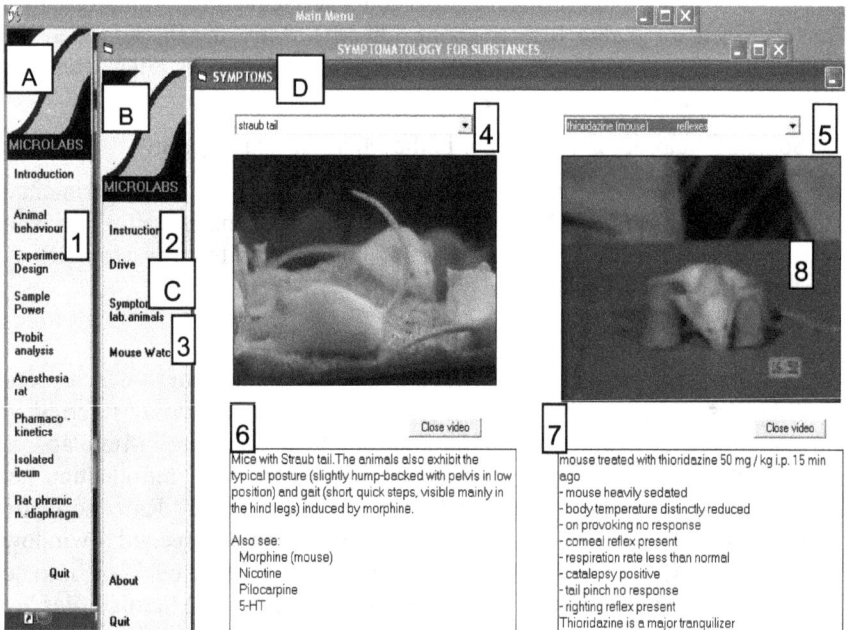

A. First Main Menu of MICROLAB

1. Click on Animal behaviour

   Allow symptoms. exe to run and Will open Second Window

B. SYMPTOMALOGY FOR SUBSTANCES

   Click on initiate and after seeing Drive box,

2. Put the drive name in which microlab is installed e.g. C, will activate tabs Symptoms lab animals and Mouse watch.

3. Click first and the third window open- D. Symptoms

With 4 boxes

4. symptom video

5. substance video

6. Information about symptoms

7. Information about substances

After going through above paragraphs and figure one can understand the worth of it as many times one can not get chance to observe all the activities in one go. Even if some who is not in favour of use of such humane approach should use it for the variety of demonstrations which may be difficult otherwise e.g. demonstration of effects of many narcotic substances like – cannabis, morphine etc, which demand many procedures to be followed to procure and use.

III.2. Mouse behaviour

After opening microlab main page, click on Mouse watch which will ask permission to run zmouse.app Allow to run by clicking yes and it will display new window to enable observing patterns of mouse behaviour in the similar way as shown above.

III.3. Experimental Design

As shown in above figures click on Experimental Design and follow the steps as shown in figure. The software is aimed at making students familiar with simulated data for designing an experiment; allow students to explore the factors which determine the number of animals to be included in a trial and student to examine and interpret a graphical display of their data. The simulation helps in planning experiments at various stages.

Choice of sample size is often the most difficult part in planning of an experiment. Five requirements for a 'good' experimental design. Experiments should:

1. be unbiased, so that comparison can be made among treatment groups;

2. Have high precision, so that if there is a true treatment effect there will be a high probability of detecting it;

3. Have a wide range of applicability, so that the results can be generalized to other sets of conditions;

4. be simple, so that no mistakes occur in their execution and subsequent statistical analysis; and

5. There should be the ability to calculate uncertainty, i.e. it should be possible to carry out a valid statistical analysis.

The simulation provides IN VIVO experiments (i.e. experiments on whole animals) in which effects are expressed either as graded responses or as quantal responses. GRADED RESPONSE is an effect that can be measured, e.g. reaction time. QUANTAL RESPONSE (All or None response) is an effect that can be counted, i.e. number of animals responding vs. number of animals not responding. The results are often expressed as ED_{50} (i.e. dose causing an effect in 50 % of the animals) or LD_{50} (i.e. dose causing the death of 50 % of the animals). For Quantal response- please refer section 5. **Probit Analysis** given below. The illustration of Hot plate method may help to understand the concept-

With the hot plate method analgesic properties of drugs, such as new synthetic drugs, isolated compounds and plant extracts, can be tested. Both, experiments measuring graded responses and experiments measuring quantal responses can be simulated in the present program. Open "Show video" for a video demonstrating the Hot Plate Method. With the simulation program Experimental Design one can explore the following questions:

Which of the drugs: morphine, pethidine (= meperdine, a synthetic analgesic belonging to the opiates) or one of the pethidine analogues has the strongest analgesic property. What are the ED_{50} values for these drugs? How many animals do one need in an experiment, for example by comparing pethidine with one of the pethidine derivatives.

The experiments can be performed by measuring the latency time (graded response), or by counting the number of animals exceeding the maximal latency time.

Exploring Graded Response

The response will be measured on a continuous scale, e.g. the period elapsed after the application of the drug (in the case of opiates in the hot plate test a period of 30 seconds is taken as 100 %). The response is due to variation.

By selecting dose and number of animals to be tested, a dose-response relation can be established. The present experiment also allows one to design an experiment with an optimal sample size, based on power determination see the topic

III.4. Sample Size and Power Determination given in next section.

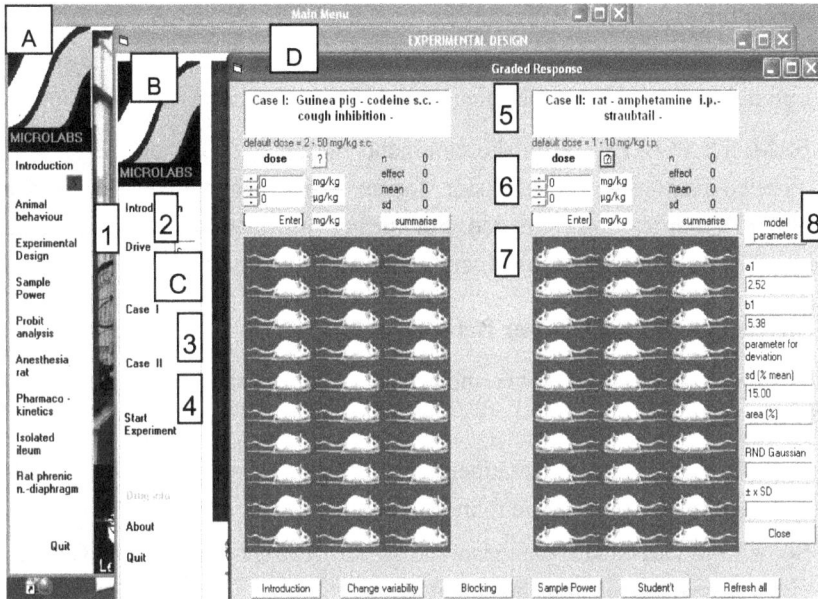

Please see similar figure, for probit Analysis
(Quantal response in same manner as above)

A. First Main Menu of MICROLAB

1. Click on Experimental Design, Allow design. exe to run and Will open Second Window B.EXPERIMENTAL DESIGN -Click on initiate and after seeing Drive box,

2. Put the drive name in which microlab is installed e.g. C, will activate tabs Case-I and Case II.

3. Click Case I and case II, Select the experiments to be performed and

4. Click on Start Experiment, New window opens- D. Graded Response.

5. shows expt selected

6. One can select Dose, Click ? to know default dose.

7. Select any no. of animals for each case and Click Summarize. The results will be summarized

8. In some experiments Model parameters can be set

9. The bottom of window has various tabs for introduction, changing variability, blocking, sample power, student t test and to refresh all data.

One can use following options for learning the experiment-

1. repeat the experiment with another dose and make a dose-response curve,
2. or one can compare the drug with an analogue drug, same dose- an optimal sample size can be calculated with the tool 'Sample power"

SAMPLE POWER- With the command button POWER on the screens for Graded responses, the precision for an experiment with a Test and a Treatment group can be estimated. For further information see III.4 Sample Size and Power Determination given below.

III. 4. Sample Size and Power Determination

The relationship between power and required number can be calculated with the tool Sample Power.

In order to compare two treatment groups the required number of subjects in each treatment group can be found as follows:

- Set with the scrollbars the mean and sd for treatment group A (= Case I), either as real values or as percentages.
- One has to decide now how much the mean of the treatment group (B) should differ from the mean of the test group, e.g. 1.5 x the sd value.
- Next select the level of significance, for example $p < 0.05$. (Since the distribution is symmetrical one should select alpha = 0.025).
- With the scrollbar the required number of animals vs. the power can be found. In general a power of 0.8 is acceptable for an experiment (see below Theory).

Example

Case I – mouse, pethidine, dose e.g. mg/kg for the analgesic effect.

The analgesic effect is based on the so-called hot-plate experiment. A mouse placed on a hot plate of 56 degrees Celsius will feel uncomfortable and starts licking its paws. The time before the animal feels uncomfortable will be delayed and is measured here as percentage of a chosen maximal delay time.

Case II – one of the analogues of pethidine, same dose.

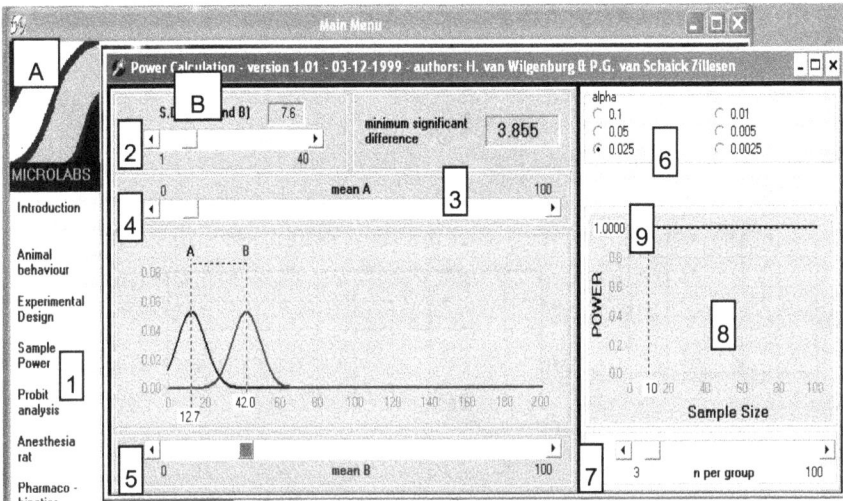

A. First Main Menu of MICROLAB

The sample Power software can be opened directly from main MICROLAB window or by clicking Sample Power in experimental Design as shown above.

1. Click on Sample Power, Allow power. exe to run and Will open Second Window B.POWER Calculation –

2. The bar allows adjusting SD of both groups under study

3. The window automatically displays min. significant diff.

4. One can adjust mean of group A

5. One can adjust mean of group A

6. Select alpha (usually 0.05)

7. Select number of subject/animal per group

8. Simulation will display the graph Sample Size Vs Power

9. With Cursor one can find values of both axes at particular point on graph.

III. 5. Probit Analysis

One can perform an experiment with different doses of a drug. To undergo the probit analyses one need to collect the following data:

The dose, n, and the percentage of animals responding after which one can obtain from the Table the corresponding probit values for the percentages.

One can calculate the ED_{50} or LD_{50} with the linear regression method as follows:

For a linear relationship $Y = A + BX$ between the log dose (X) and the probits (Y), the parameters A (Y-intercept) and B (regression coefficient or slope) can be estimated with the method of least squares or one may refer the chapter-11 for computer application in data analyses.

Verify your outcome by clicking the "Probit analysis" button.

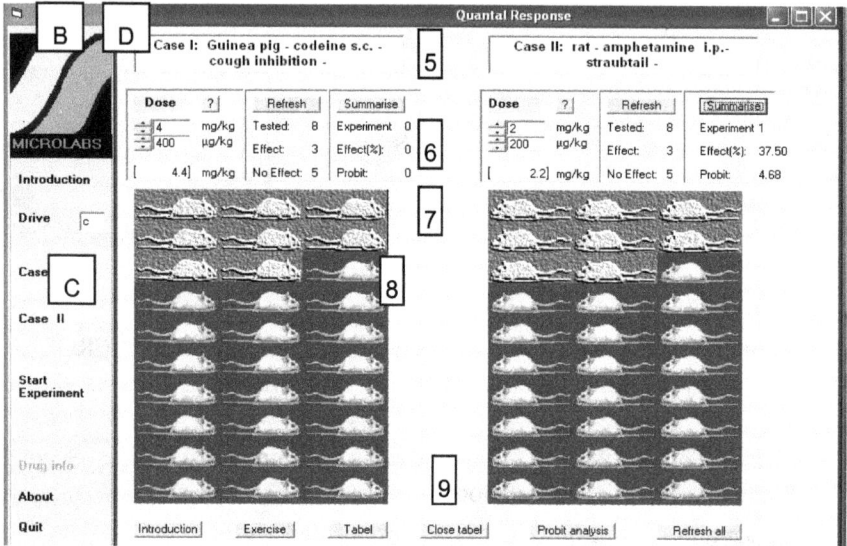

Please see similar figure, for Experimental Design (Graded response) for initial steps.

The steps are similar as shown above in **EXPERIMENTAL DESIGN,** instead click B.**Probit Analysis**

For starting-Steps- 1-9 are similar to earlier figure for experimental design except 8 where one can see numbers of animals selected for study.

After giving the dose in suggested dose range, it will show results out of given animals in how many animals effect was observed. After clicking summarize tab (7), the data in form of % effect, and Probit will appear.

One can repeat experiment with different dose and animals as per wish and every time the data obtained will be used for plotting graph when the tab Probit analysis is clicked.

It will provide the straight line from which LD or ED values can be obtained.

III. 6. Anaesthesia of the rat

The simulation shows induction of anaesthesia with different anaesthetics in different animals. It gives choice of few anaesthetics and one can observe the effect of same after administration through the route suggested. It provides VDOs also showing the administration techniques and reflexes in animal. One can easily understand the administration technique, dosing, effect of dose on various parameters like onset, duration of anaesthesia; heart rate, ECG and respiration.

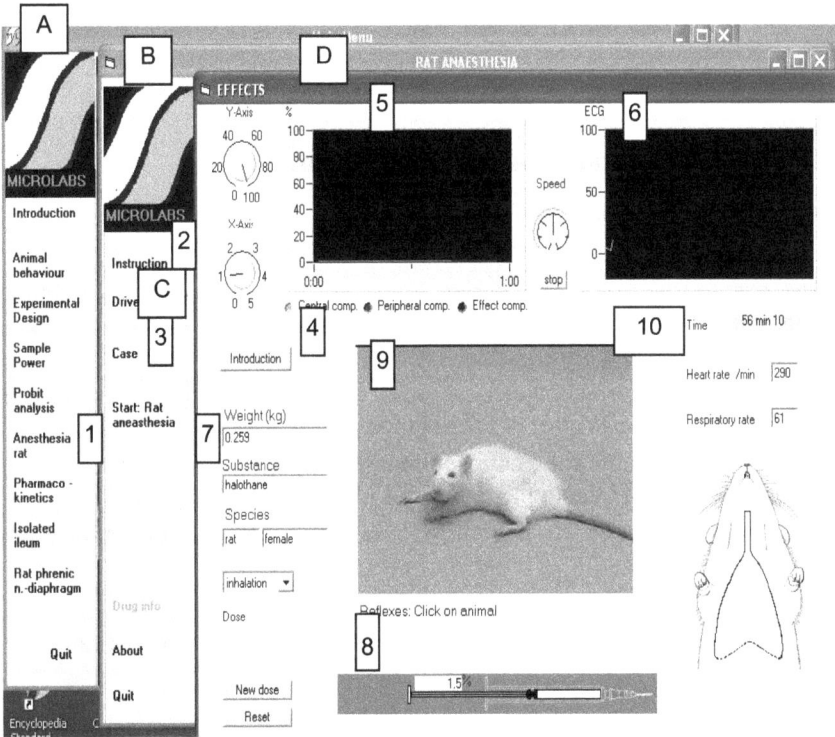

A.   First Main Menu of MICROLAB

1.   Click on Anaesthesia Rat, Allow ANESTH~1. exe to run and Will open Second Window B.RAT ANAESTHETIA -Click on initiate and after seeing Drive box,

2.   Put the drive name in which microlab is installed e.g. C, will activate tabs Case

3.   Click Case and Select the anaesthesia. And click start. This will open tab D. EFFCTS.

4.   Read instructions

5. The monitor will show the concentration of drugs in different compartment
6. The changes in ECG during anaesthesia can be observed
7. Select the weight of animal, animal details, substance (anaesthetic agent) mode of administration, Dose (one can refer the usual dose mentioned above the syringe)
8. Click Apply near Syringe.
9. This window shows many VDOs that can demonstrate from technique of administration to various signs. The beauty of the simulation is that it matches all the parameter with time.
10. Shows time elapsed, heart rate and respiratory rate at given time.
11. The animation shows pattern of respiration.

III. 7. Human case studies and pharmacokinetics

This software simulation is aimed-

1. to illustrate some of the aspects of pharmacokinetics,
2. to ensure that one can derive some of the basic pharmacokinetic parameters from curves relating plasma concentration to time after administration of a drug,
3. to show how correct choice of dose and dosage regimen can ensure appropriate plasma concentrations are achieved,
4. to demonstrate how the pharmacokinetic behaviour of drugs varies from agent to agent and the implications this has for drug therapy, and,
5. to give practise in finding and retrieving specific information from literature sources.

The computer Simulation model allows the person to generate data relating the plasma concentration of drugs to the time after administration.

This data can be obtained

1. as a screen display using linear arithmetic concentration (y) and time (x) axes or,
2. as a screen display using a log10 concentration (y) and arithmetic time (x) axes.

Measurements can be taken directly from the screen displays which are largely self-explanatory. Note the scale and units on the concentration axis. The program chooses an appropriate scale on which to plot the graphs but one can change the concentration scale by specifying the top value for the scale if one wish. This sometimes makes it easier to compare a set of graphs (since they have a common y-axis scale) or it can be used to magnify the lower part of a graphical display showing a large sharp peak of concentration. The data can also be obtained in numerical form which one can plot oneself. Note that it is not necessary to plot every point for which data are given to obtain an adequate graph relating plasma concentration to time.

The upper (maximum therapeutic) and lower (minimum effective) plasma concentrations for each drug are displayed numerically at the top of the screen display. If these upper and lower concentrations fall within the scale of the graphical presentation they are also displayed as lines across the screen at the appropriate concentration level. Note that these are guide line concentrations only. In the program these concentrations have fixed values but in practise they will vary from subject to subject and will also depend ON THE THERAPEUTIC USE OF THE DRUG. For example the minimum effective concentration of aspirin depends on whether it is being used as a minor analgesic (headache) or as an anti-inflammatory agent (rheumatoid arthritis). For antibacterial drugs like ampicillin the effective concentration will depend on the sensitivity of the organism. In vitro minimum inhibitory concentrations may be as low as 0.02 µg/ml (streptococcus pneumoniae) or as high as 500 µg/ml (β lactamase producing H. influenzae).

What is a toxic level may depend on -

1. the duration for which tissues are exposed to a concentration of the drug;
2. the nature and seriousness of the toxic effect in relation to the likely benefits of treatment;
3. the particular aspect of toxicity considered;
4. the proportion of patients that experience toxicity.

Gentamicin for example can produce vestibular damage (tinnitus, vertigo), deafness (less often) or nephrotoxicity. The proportion of patients exhibiting these effects at a plasma concentration of say 15 µg/ml is very different and depends on the duration of exposure to the drug.

Toxicity can also be affected by the degree of protein binding (reduced in hypoalbuminaemia, uraemia or by interactions with other drugs). Allergic reactions can occur at any concentration of drug. The effective and toxic concentrations shown are therefore GUIDE-LINES only.

The model assumes that all drugs given by intravenous injection are administered as a bolus over a few seconds. This will produce a very high initial peak plasma concentration. In practice many drugs are given iv by a slow injection over 2-3 minutes and this produces a lower initial plasma concentration. Note also that oral dosage forms may be available which release the drug slowly, quickly or over a sustained period. Clearly the characteristics of the particular dosage form used will influence the shape of the plasma concentration-time plot.

The program will ask the user for certain information about the subject in whom the measurements are being made (e.g. normal? liver failure?) and about the dosage regimen (e.g. size of dose? frequency of dosing?). These can be set as one's wish or according to the instructions one have been given. Note that the duration of the investigation specifies the time period (hours) over which measurements of plasma concentration of drug will be taken. Allow sufficient time for steady-state to be established if using multiple dose regimens or for plasma concentrations to fall to very low levels if single doses are used.

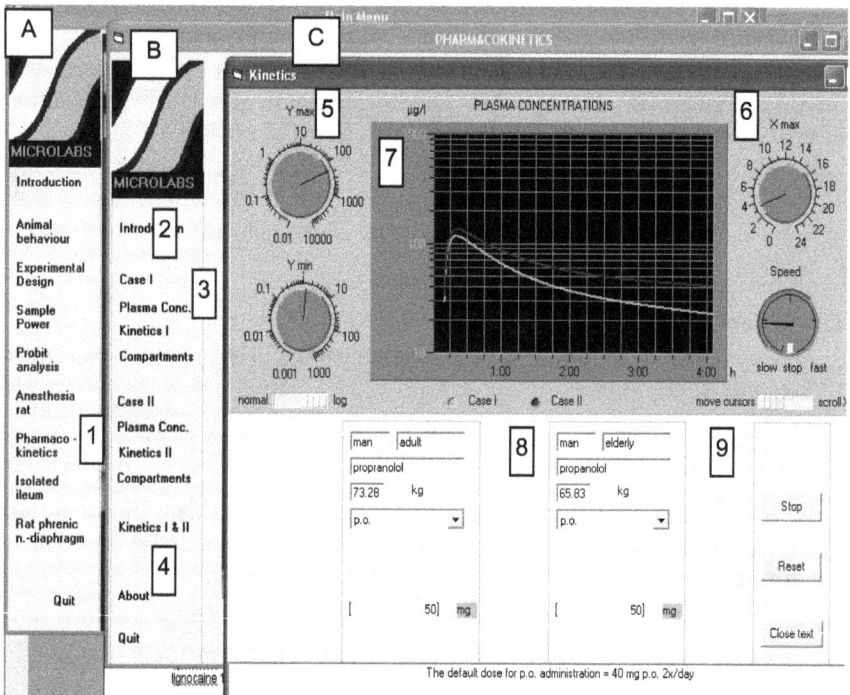

A. First Main Menu of MICROLAB

1. Click on Pharmacokinetics, Allow kinetics.exe to run and Will open Second Window B.PHARMACOKINETICS -Click on initiate and after seeing Drive box,

2. One can see introduction

3. Click Case I and case II- will provide several options like species and for each species drug and/or condition. Select the desired and click confirm

   Select the parameters to be observed by clicking Plasma Conc. (will show Plasma Conc. of given case), Kinetics-I and II (Kinetics of each case separately) and Compartments. (movement of drug in different compartments i.e. concentration in each compartment at given time.

4. Click on Kinetic I & II- New window opens- C. Kinetics
5. The knobs allow the change graph height i.e. Y-scale, scale divisions and type of paper normal or semi log.
6. The knobs allow the change graph speed & X-scale,
7. Displays real time graph
8. One can confirm the species and case selected, select the route and dose (clue for default can be seen at bottom obtained after clicking question mark)
9. The panel allows starting, stopping and resetting the experiment. Second dose may be added at any time to see the impact of second dose.

EXAMPLES OF WORK SCHEDULES

1. ROUTES OF ADMINISTRATION. Generate plasma concentration-time plots for single doses of 500 mg of ampicillin given iv and orally (6 h duration), ampicillin given as an intravenous infusion (42 mg/hr given over 12 h) and for diazepam 20 mg given iv and orally (24 h duration).

   NB. Ampicillin is a weak acid drug with a pKa = 2.5.

   For each route and drug derive and tabulate:-

   (a) the maximum plasma concentration achieved
   (b) the time for an effective concentration to be established
   (c) the duration for which it is exceeded
   (d) the time for which maximum therapeutic levels are exceeded.

2. BIOAVAILABILITY.-Generate plasma concentration-time plots of 12 h duration for 10 mg and for 500 mg ampicillin given orally and by iv injection and for 10 mg of diazepam given orally and iv (96 h duration). Measure the area under the curves.

   For each dose tabulate:-
   (a) the maximum plasma concentration achieved
   (b) the time for which a therapeutic concentration was maintained
   (c) the area under the curve.

3. BASIC PHARMACOKINETIC PARAMETERS (A).-Generate a plasma concentration-time plot of 96 h duration for 25 mg diazepam given iv in a normal subject. Obtain the numerical data either displayed on the screen or as hardcopy from the printer. Plot a graph of log1O plasma concentration or log (ln; natural log) plasma concentration on the y axis

against time (x axis). [Note that it makes a difference which one user choose; $\ln X = 2.303 \log_{10} X$]. One may use semi log paper if it is available and one is familiar with its use.

4. BASIC PHARMACOKINETIC PARAMETERS (A)-Generate a plasma concentration-time plot of 24 h duration for 100 mg gentamicin given iv in a normal subject and in a subject with kidney failure. One may need to repeat the plots over a longer period to make sure plasma concentration reach very low levels (i.e. all the drug removed).

5. REPEATED DOSING (A).-Generate plasma concentration-time plots of 180 h duration for 40, 75, 150, 300 and 600 mg of quinidine given orally every 6 h and for phenytoin 20, 40, 60, 80, 100, 120, 150 mg given orally every 8 h for 240 h. Estimate the steady-state concentration achieved and the time required to achieve it at each dose level. Tabulate the data.

6. REPEATED DOSING (B).-Generate plasma concentration-time plots of 240 h duration for oral administration of digoxin 0.5 mg every 24 h, paracetamol 600 mg every 4 h, diazepam 10 mg every 12 h and ampicillin 500 mg every 6 h. For each drug estimate the steady-state concentration achieved, the time required to achieve it and the peak-trough variation Express the peak-trough variation as a percentage of the therapeutic window for each drug.

7. REPEATED DOSING (C).-Generate plasma concentration-time plots of 120 h duration for oral administration of paracetamol every 2, 4, 8, 12 and 24 h choosing a dose for each dose interval so that the dose rate per 24 h period is the same and equal to 3600 mg per 24 h.

8. LOADING DOSE.-Generate plasma concentration-time plots for digoxin 0.1, 0.27 0.4 and 0.6 mg given every 12 h orally for 300 h. Tabulate for each dosage regimen the steady-state concentrations achieved, the time required to reach steady-state and the time required for effective and/or toxic levels to be achieved.

9. IV INFUSIONS.-Generate plasma concentration-time plots for an iv infusion of lignocaine at 100 mg/hr for 48 h and for administration of lignocaine 100 mg, iv every hour for 48 h.

Tabulate for each dosage regimen:-

(a) the time required to reach steady-state

(b) the average steady-state plasma concentration achieved [Note that one will need to think about what to take as the average plasma concentration and to justify the way one have chosen to estimate this value.]

(c) (iv bolus only) the size of the peak-to-trough difference.

8. Guinea pig ileum *in vitro*

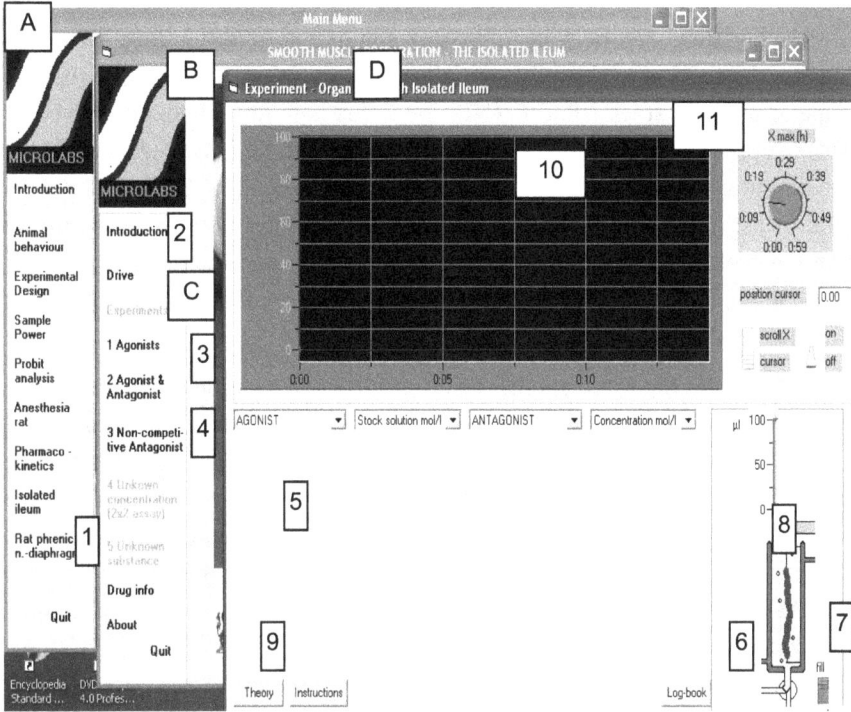

A. First Main Menu of MICROLAB

1. Click on Experimental Design, Allow ileum. exe to run and Will open Second Window B.Smooth Muscle Preparation -Click on initiate and after seeing Drive box,

2. Put the drive name in which microlab is installed e.g. C, will activate tabs below.

3. Before selecting any option on the window one can see the VDO by opting for same.

4. Click on any tab 1agonist-3Non competitive antagonist. Will open New window D. Experiment- Organ Bath with isolated ileum

5. Allows selecting agonist, antagonists and their concentrations.

6. Organ bath with tissue and transducer.

7. Knob allowing filling and emptying of organ bath.

8. Micropipette allowing administration the dose of selected substance.

9. The bottom of window has various tabs for theory, instruction and log book.

10. The monitor showing response to the drug.

11. The knobs allow to change settings of the speed of physiograph

Methodology

Following steps can help in using this simulation in better way. Select an agonist (usually acetylcholine initially), -select its stock solution, -fill the pipette with the stock solution (NB. the organ bath has a bath volume of 10 ml). Apply the agonist; the batch concentration will be indicated, - 'wash' the preparation by emptying and refilling the organ bath, -switch off the recorder and measure the contraction (in mm) by moving the cursor. Keep record of the concentration of the agonist in the organ bath and the amplitude of the contraction. (One can make use of the Excel-sheet. Close text. Right click the field and select 'open'). See Graph5.

Administer the same agonist again in the same or another concentration. One can increase the concentration with steps of a factor 2, for example 10, 20, 50, 100, 200, etc nmol/l (1 nanomol/l = 1E- 9 mol/l). Repeat the experiment at any concentration at least 3 times. Plot the experimental data on graphics paper and draw the best fitting concentration-effect curve; put the bath concentration on the abscise and on the ordinate the contraction height or the percentage of the maximal contraction; (see Fig. 3 and Graph1 by clicking figures). Find the EC50. Plot the same data on semi-logarithmic paper and draw a log concentration-effect curve (see Fig. 4 and Graph2).

Finally one can make a Line weaver-Burk-plot (use only the data obtained from concentrations close to the EC50). Calculate the reciprocal values (1/effect and 1/concentration) and plot the results on graphics paper; draw a straight line and find the parameters Emax and Ka (see Fig. 5 and Graph 3). Compare the Kd with the value in the drug info section.

The experiment can now be repeated with another agonist. Take at least two other agonists (suggestion: furmethide and angiotensin). If other students do the same for some other drugs, one can compare the results.

- select first an agonist (suggestion; begin with acetylcholine) and make a concentration-effect curve as one have made in the former section.
- select an antagonist (suggestion take atropine in a concentration of 1E-8 mol/l) and repeat the experiment with the former agonist in the presence of the antagonist then draw the concentration-effect curve in the same graph. 'Wash' the antagonist and repeat the former procedure for at least two other concentrations of the same antagonist. Find the pA2 with the aid of an Arunlakshana-Schild plot. (see Fig. 7a and 7b and Graph4).

III. 9. Phrenic nerve-diaphragm *in vitro*

The software explains many basics behind the experiment. It also shows the figure of assembly set up for the experiment.

IV.   WINSIMS - Strathclyde Pharmacology Simulations (Author Dr.John Dempster, Dept of Physiology & Pharmacology, Institute for Biomedical Sciences, University of Strathclyde, Glasgow, G4 0NR, UK)

The Strathclyde Pharmacology Simulations package is a suite of programs simulating pharmacological experiments on isolated tissues or whole animals. A range of drugs in varying concentrations can be applied and the effects observed. The programs will run under Windows 95 or later. It contains following softwares- Anaesthetised Cat, Pithed Rat, Nerve-Muscle Preparation, Neuromuscular junction Electrophysiology

IV. 1. The Virtual Cat

The Virtual Cat is a simulation of the anaesthetised cat experiment - a whole animal preparation which is widely used as a tool for screening the actions of new pharmaceutical compounds on the cardiovascular and skeletal muscle systems. The simulation allows observing the traces of blood pressure, heart rate, skeletal muscle and nictitating membrane twitches on the screen, to apply a variety of different drugs and to observe their effects.

The Anaesthetised Cat Preparation is simulation of experimental set up as given below-

Adult cat is anaesthetised by intraperitoneal injection of a chloralose + pentabarbitone mixture, tracheally intubated, and artificially ventilated. A cannula is inserted into the left brachial vein and used to administer drugs. Arterial blood pressure is measured via a cannula inserted into the right carotid artery and connected to a pressure transducer. The heart rate is derived from this blood pressure signal. The vagus nerve is exposed at the neck (but not cut) and hooked over stimulation electrodes. This nerve innervates the heart, via the ganglion (G) shown. Stimulation causes a reduction in heart rate. The cervical sympathetic nerve is exposed at the neck (ligated preganglionically) and a stimulation electrode attached. This nerve innervates the nictitating membrane over the eye of cat, via a nicotinic ganglion. The nictitating membrane is attached to a tension transducer. Stimulation of the nerve causes a contraction of the nictitating membrane. One end of the tibialis muscle (fast type skeletal muscle), in the leg of the cat, is dissected free and attached to a tension transducer. The sciatic nerve is exposed and attached to stimulation electrodes. Stimulation of the nerve causes a muscle twitch. The muscle is innervated via nicotinic receptors at the neuromuscular junction.

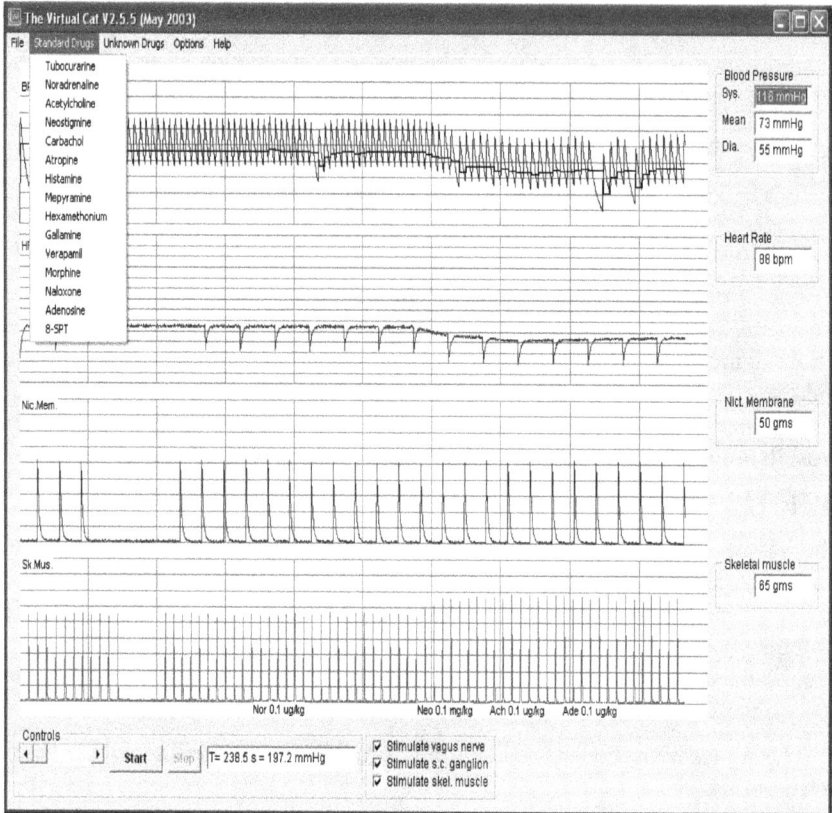

Using the simulation

1. Select New Cat from the File menu, to clear the chart.
2. Click the Start button to start the chart recorder running.
3. To inject a drug into the cats circulation :-
   (a) Select a drug from the Standard Drugs menu.
   (b) Select the required dose from the list of doses.
   (c) Click Inject Drug button to add the drug.
4. One can make quantitative measurements from the traces by moving the mouse cursor over the trace and noting the value in the readout at the bottom of the screen.
5. One can add as many doses and/or drugs as necessary. When one has finished the experiment, click the Stop button to stop the chart.
6. To print out a hard copy of the traces shown on the screen, Select Print from the File menu.

7. When one has completed an experiment, can save it to a storage file by selecting Save Cat ... from the File menu. (To re-load an experiment, select Load Cat ...).

8. To exit from the simulation program, select Exit from the File menu.

The basics behind the simulations

The vagus nerve releases acetylcholine and acts via muscarinic cholinoceptors (mAChR) on the heart to slow heart rate and reduce cardiac force.

* The baroreceptor reflex. Baroreceptors within the CNS when stimulated by high arterial presssure increase the nerve activity along the vagus depressing heart rate and force

* The accelerans nerves releases noradrenaline and acts via B-adrenoceptors (bAdr) on the heart to increase heart rate and contractile force.

* Both the vagus and accelerans nerves act indirectly via ganglia. Synaptic transmission at the ganglia is by neuronal nicotinic cholinoceptors (nAChR).

* Mu-Opioid and adenosine (A1) receptors are present on the presynaptic nerve endings of both the vagus and accelerans nerves and act to depress transmitter release.

* Heart muscle also has adenosine (A1) receptors which cause a reduction in heart rate and force in response to circulating adenosine.

  Smooth muscle in the walls of arteries act to constrict the vessels. The blood vessels are innervated by sympathetic nerves, via nicotinic ganglia and are also sensitive to drugs in the circulation.

* The sympathetic nerves release noradrenaline which acts upon α-adrenoceptors in the smooth muscle to cause vasoconstriction which increases blood pressure.

* Circulating acetylcholine can produce vasodilatation by acting upon muscarinic receptors on endothelial cells to release vasodilators.

* Circulating adenosine can produce vasodilatation by acting upon adenosine (A1) receptors in the smooth muscle.

* Circulating histamine can produce vasodilatation by acting upon histamine (H1) receptors.

  The nictitating membrane is a protective membrane which can be drawn over the cats eye. It contains smooth muscle and is indirectly innervated by the superior cervical nerve. Stimulation of the pre-ganglionic nerve causes the membrane to contract.

* The smooth muscle has α-adrenoceptors which respond to noradrenaline released by the nerve.

*   The post-ganglionic nerve terminals which release noradrenaline have pre-synaptic Mu-opioid (uOpR) and adenosine (A_1) receptors which act to depress transmitter release.
*   The superior cervical ganglion is a neuronal nicotinic synapse.
    The tibialis muscle is a fast skeletal muscle, innervated directly via the sciatic nerve. Stimulation of the nerve produces a muscle twitch.
*   The nerve releases acetylcholine which acts upon nicotinic cholinoceptors (AchR) at the neuromuscular junction to cause a muscle twitch.
*   The muscle does not respond to circulating acetylcholine with a contracture since depolarization block occurs (a combination of sodium channel inactivation and receptor desensitization) in response to the slow and prolonged application of Ach.

IV. 2. The Virtual Rat

The Virtual Rat is a simulation of a pithed rat experimental preparation for investigating the actions of drugs on the heart and cardiovascular system. "Pithing" refers to the destruction of spinal cord pathways, severing all the nerve connections between the brain and the cardiovascular system. This greatly simplifies the interpretation of experimental results by removing the central baroreceptor reflexes. The simulation allows observing traces of blood pressure, left ventricular pressure, venous pressure, heart rate and contractile force on a simulated chart recorder, to apply a variety of different drugs, and to observe their effects.

The Rat Cardiovascular System Preparation is simulation of experimental set up as given below-

A rat is anaesthetised and artificially ventilated. Three cannulae are inserted into the femoral artery, vein and the left ventricle of the heart. The arterial cannula is connected to a pressure transducer to measure arterial blood pressure. Traces of arterial blood pressure (ABP) and heart rate (HR), computed from ABP, are recorded on the chart recorder. The left ventricular cannula is connected to a second pressure transducer and used to produce a trace of left ventricular pressure (LVP). A measure of the contractile force of the heart (HF) is derived from the LVP.

The venous cannula is connected to a third pressure transducer and used to produce a trace of central venous blood pressure (VBP). Drugs can also be injected into the animal via the venous cannula. A specially designed pithing rod can be passed down the spinal cord of the animal destroying all nerve connections with the brain, and hence disabling the central blood pressure reflexes associated with the carotid artery baroreceptors.

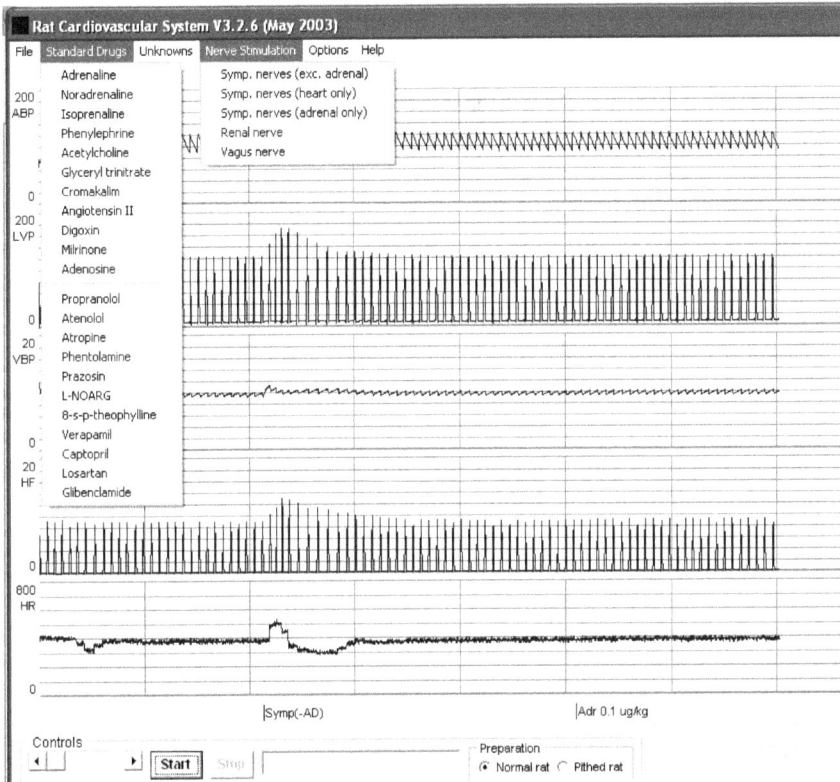

Using the simulation

1. Select New Rat from the File menu, to clear the chart.

2. Click the Start button to start the chart recorder running.

3. To inject a drug into the animal's circulation :

   (a) Select a drug from the Standard Drugs menu.

   (b) Select the required dose from the list of doses.

   (c) Click Inject Drug button to add the drug.

4. One can make quantitative measurements from the traces by moving the mouse cursor over the trace and noting the value in the readout at the bottom of the screen.

5. One can add as many doses and/or drugs as necessary. When one has finished the experiment, click the Stop button to stop the chart.

6. To print out a hard copy of the traces shown on the screen, Select Print from the File menu.

7. When one have completed an experiment it can be saved to a storage file by selecting Save Rat ... from the File menu. (To re-load an experiment, select Load Rat ...).

8. To exit from the simulation program, select Exit from the File menu.

IV. 3. The Virtual Rat

The Virtual Rat is a simulation of the rat phrenic nerve-hemidiaphragm preparation - a robust in vitro preparation which has been widely used in the study the actions of neuromuscular blocking and reversal agents, and other drugs which affect neuromuscular transmission.

The hemidiaphraghm is a large, focally innervated, respiratory skeletal muscle, composed of fast-type muscle fibres. Neurotransmission is mediated by nicotinic cholinoceptors. Electrical stimulation of the phrenic nerve evokes fast, shorting-lasting muscle twitches.

The Rat Phrenic Nerve - Hemidiaphragm Preparation

A rat (0.5 Kg) is killed by anaesthetising it with 100% CO_2 (a rapid and fairly painless procedure). The rib cage is opened and the phrenic nerve and triangular-shaped hemidiaphragm is removed and placed into an organ bath containing Kreb's solution, bubbled with 95%O_2/5%CO_2, and maintained at 32C by a surrounding water bath. As shown in the diagram, the base of the muscle is attached to a support and the tendon attached to a tension transducer. The nerve is looped through a stimulation electrode and another electrode is placed directly upon the muscle. Drugs are applied directly into the bath. When required, drugs can be washed out, by flushing it out with new Kreb's solution.

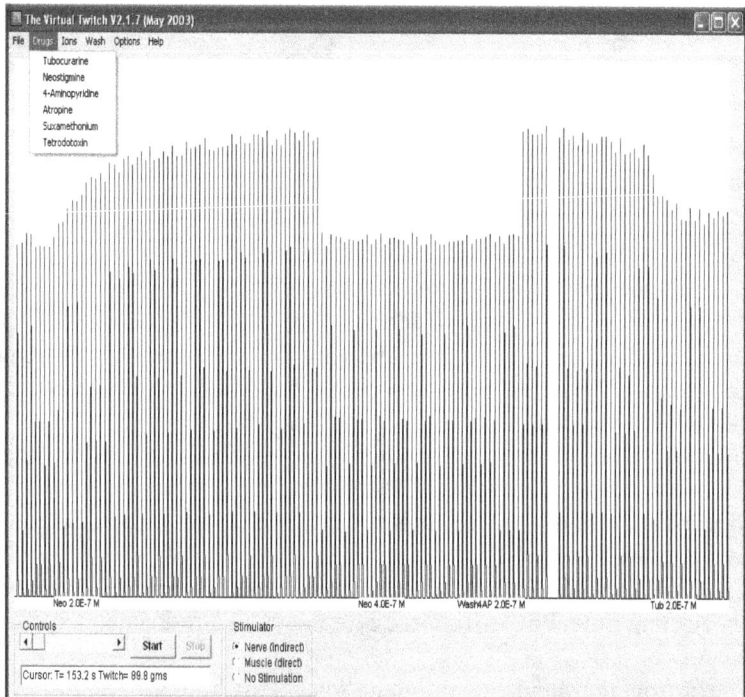

Using the simulation

1. Select New Rat from the File menu, to clear the chart.

2. Click the Start button to start the chart recorder running.

3. To inject a drug into the cats circulation :

    (a)   Select a drug from the Drugs menu.

    (b)   Select the required dose from the list of doses.

    (c)   Click Inject Drug button to add the drug.

4. One can make quantitative measurements from the traces by moving the mouse cursor over the trace and noting the value in the readout at the bottom of the screen.

5. One can add as many doses and/or drugs as necessary. When one has finished experiment, click the Stop button to stop the chart.

6. To print out a hard copy of the traces shown on the screen, Select Print from the File menu.

7. When one have completed an experiment it can be saved to a storage file by selecting Save Rat ... from the File menu. (To re-load an experiment, select Load Rat ...).

8. To exit from the simulation program, select Exit from the File menu.

IV. 4. The Virtual NMJ

The Virtual NMJ is a simulation of an experiment recording the electrical potentials associated with neuromuscular transmission at the skeletal neuromuscular junction.

Electrophysiological measurements provide a more direct insight into the mechanisms of neuromuscular transmission than the measurement of muscle tension. Bernard Katz's studies of the endplate potential, for instance, lead to the discovery of the quantal nature of transmitter release and further use of the techniques have revealed the precise mechanism of action of many of the drugs that affect neuromuscular transmission.

The simulation allows one to observe the muscle action potential (AP) and endplate potentials (EPPs) evoked by either nerve stimulation or by direct current stimulation of the muscle fibre. The effects of a variety of drugs and of changes to ionic composition of the extracellular solution on the AP and EPPs can be studied.

Nerve-muscle preparation

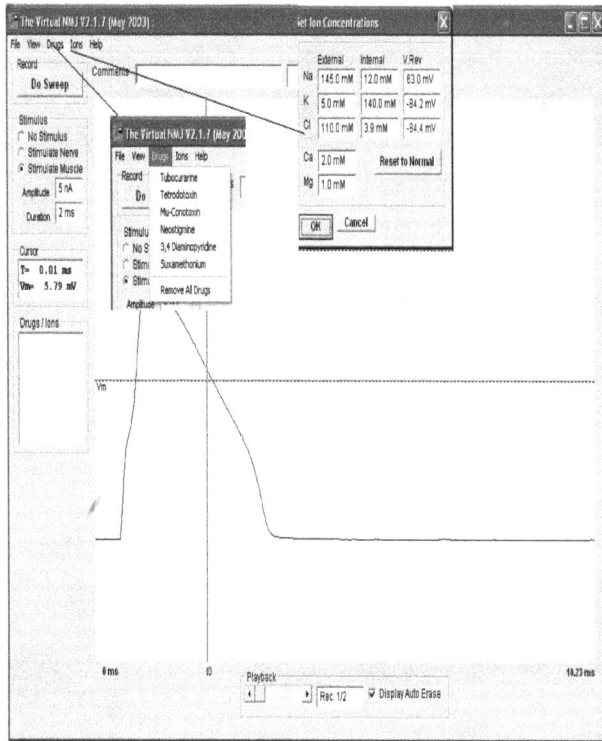

Using the simulation

1. Select New Experiment from the File menu to start a new experiment. The preparation is set up initially with no drugs and a Krebs solution with normal ionic concentrations.

2. An experiment consists of a series of recording sweeps, acquired under different drugs and/or ionic concentration conditions. To initiate a recording sweep, click the Do Sweep button.

3. To add a drug to the preparation (or change its concentration) : (a) Select a drug from the Drugs menu, (b) Enter the required concentration (M), (c) Click the OK button to add the drug, (d) Click the Do Sweep button to see the effect of the drug.

4. To change the ionic composition of the extracellular solution : (a) Select the Ions menu option, (b) Change the required ionic concentration (mM), (c) Click the OK button to change the concentration. (d) Click the Do Sweep button to see the effect of the concentration change.

5. One can inspect each sweep that one has recorded by using the Playback scroll bar to redisplay that record on the screen. One can magnify the display by double-clicking on the display to get the Magnification dialog box. If one want to superimpose a number of records, un-check the Display Auto-Erase box.

6. One can make quantitative measurements from the traces by dragging the grey vertical cursor over the trace and noting the value in the cursor readout box. Measurements are made relative to the grey horizontal baseline cursor which can be repositioned by dragging it up or down. (0 mV is indicated by a dotted blue line).

7. To print out a hard copy of the traces shown on the screen, Select Print from the File menu.

8. To save the experiment, select Save Experiment from the File menu and enter the name of a data file. One can re-load this experiment at a later date using Load Experiment.

9. To exit from the simulation program, select Exit from the File menu.

The hemidiaphragm muscle with attached phrenic nerve is dissected from a rat and pinned out in flat dish. Oxygenated (95% O2, 5% CO2) Kreb's solution is superfused in a constant stream over the preparation. The dish is placed on a microscope stage and a fine (tip diameter < 0.1 micron) glass micropipette electrode inserted in the endplate region of a muscle fibre.

The electrode is connected via a microelectrode amplifier to an oscilloscope, displaying the intracellular membrane potential of the muscle fibre.

The muscle can be stimulated in either of two ways.

1. DIRECTLY - by injecting a small current into the muscle fibre via the recording electrode. The amplitude and duration of the stimulus current can be set within the simulation.

2. INDIRECTLY - by stimulating the phrenic nerve via platinum wire electrode.

Drugs are applied via the Kreb's solution flowing over the preparation, whose ionic composition can also be changed.

V. PharmaTutor (Author : Dr.Daniel Keller, Institute of Pharmacology, University of Zurich, Switzerland) PharmaTutor is a computer program to assist the teaching of an introductory course in pharmacology. It was designed to make the teaching of pharmacology attractive and lively without the use of animals in experiments. The program consists of five parts, each one designed to be a self-contained practical class exercise that can be completed in relatively short time (20 to 25 minutes). In a typical practical class, students circulate in small groups around a series of exercises, some of which are from PharmaTutor and others of which are written exercises, calculations, or discussion sessions. The five experiments of PharmaTutor are: Pharmacokinetic Simulations, Blood Pressure and Catecholamines, Blood Pressure and Acetylcholine, Dose Response curve using Smooth muscle in an Organ Bath, Neuro-muscular transmission.

V. 1. Pharmacokinetics

This simulation shows changes in plasma concentration of given agent through given route of administration in various clinical situations like renal insufficiency. This CAL can help to teach / learn the basics of Pharmacokinetics.

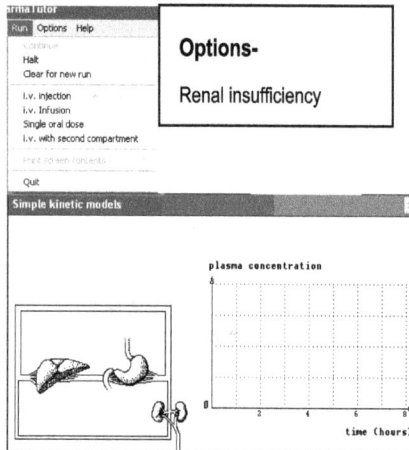

V. 2. Blood Pressure and Catacholamines and

V. 3. Blood Pressure and Acetyl Choline-

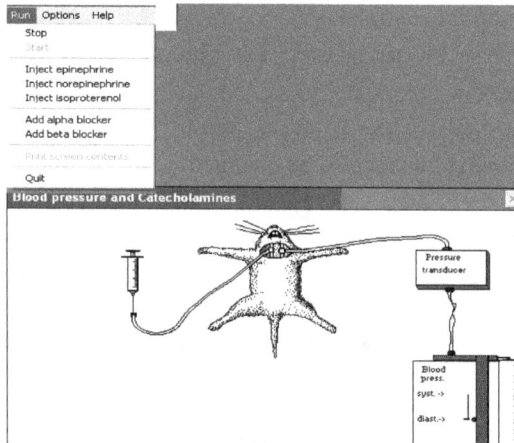

Both simulations show the effects of catecholamines and Acetyl Choline on blood pressure of animal (rat). In run bar many options can be seen for administration of various catecholamines. Similar options can be found for Ach like administration of small dose/ large dose of   Ach, administration of atropine and ganglion blocker. The effects can be seen on the paper chart moving away from the recorder.

V. 4. Dose-Response Curve

This simulation demonstrates effects of various agonists and antagonists on the given tissue. The values of response can be observed on the recorder (Converter and display unit). The dose range can be adjusted from 10^{-7} to 10^{-3} by clicking on the scale. One can add agonist or antagonist in the bath and the response can be seen with or without giving washings.

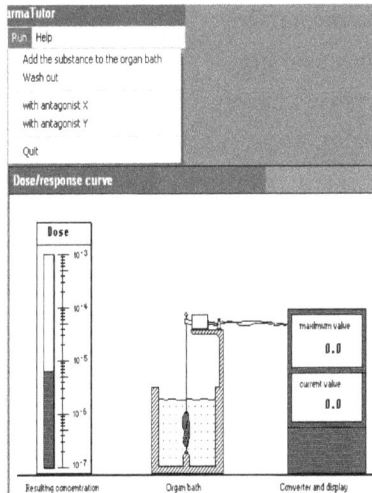

V. 5. Neuro-Muscular Transmission

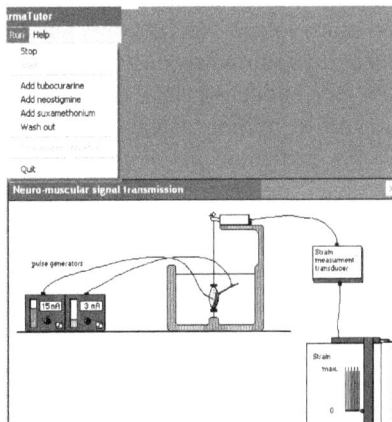

The simulations shows the effects of various agents acting on Neuro-muscular junction on the skeletal muscle preparation. It also gives option of washing the drug out.

Some URLs from where one can get information about CAL resources-

Digires: Digital Resources for Trainers - www.digires. co.uk

WINSIM, University of Strathclyde-> http://www.strath. ac.uk/Department s/PhysPharm/

Sheffield BioScience Programs http://www.sheffbp. co.uk

Pharma-CAL-ogy British Pharmacological Society www.bps.ac.uk-http://www.bps. ac.uk/site/ cms/contentCateg oryView.asp? category= 240

Biosoft www.biosoft. Com

InterNiche www.interniche. Org

AVAR database www.avar.org

EuRCA database www.eurca.org

NORINA database http://oslovet. veths.no/ NORINA/

CoAcS http://www.coacs. com/software/ bespoke_software /default. htm http://www.coacs. com/software/ published_ titles/pharmacol ogy_menu. Htm

IAUPHAR http://www.iuphar. org/sections/ teaching/ t_resources. Html

IndPharNet www.indphar.org or

http://www.ampiweb.org/indphar/sware.htm

Important Note: As mentioned in the text above, the attempt is made to introduce some of the freely available softwares that can be used for initial introduction to the subject and reinforcement of knowledge. No attempt is made to give information about the paid softwares / simulation, how so ever good these may be. Further it is reiterated that actual conduction is the best tool and no simulation can replace the learning through it but at the same time it must be noted that these simulations are of great value at place where resources do not allow to conduct variety of experiments (There may be plenty of such places) and to minimise fear, stigma in students and undue sacrifices of animals. As explained in previous chapter these CALs form important part in alternatives attempted towards humane approach.

9

Bioassays

Bio assay term is derived from two words. Bio- biological, related to living organisms and assay- means to measure the concentration of active substance/s in a given sample. Thus Bioassay can be defined as the estimation of the potency[1] of an active agent or detection and measurement of the concentration[2] of the biologically active substance present in a given sample (mostly from natural sources) using living biological material as mode (assay medium). Here biological material means whole organism i.e animal, micro-organism etc or organs, tissues, cells and considering the growth of biotechnology receptors, proteins like molecular targets of living system tissues. It is also defined by wikipedia as- It is the comparable estimation of the nature, constitution or potency of the active principles with that of the standard drug, by means of the reaction on a living matter such as whole animal, isolated tissue or organism.

Principles of Bioassay: Burn and Dale led down several principles for bioassays-

1. All bioassays must be comparable against a standard drug or preparation- The standard substances here means that the substances of which activity is known and assured if used as prescribed by the agency responsible to maintain these standards. Internationally the standards of drugs are maintained and recommended by the Expert Committee of the Biological Standardization of W.H.O. They represent the fixed units of activity (definite weight of preparation) for drugs. In India, various Government agencies like Central Drug

---

[1]Potency Measurement- Measurement of activity of active principle/s. Usually measured if the single compound may exhibit variations in activity or presense of multiple active components in the sample making it irrational to measure the concentrations of individual compounds. e.g. Extracts containing multiple agents like digitalis extract or thyroid extract containing T_3 and T_4 etc.

[2] Concentration Measurement- The measurement of amount of active principle. Usually when activity depends upon single active substance.

Research Institute, Lucknow, Central Drug Research Laboratory, Calcutta, etc are maintaining standard drugs. Further, the reference standard must owe its activity to the principle for which the sample is being bioassayed.

2. Standard drug and new drug, as far as possible, should be identical to each other- This will make easy for the assay as any point on dose –response curve can give the concentration of unknown (test) sample.

3. As far as possible during bioassays Activity assayed should be the activity of interest i.e. the therapeutic activity to be measured- The therapeutic effect to be compare instead of effects like hypoglycaemic convulsions in animals or digitalis bioassay using chick embryonic heart. The better should be to observe the therapeutic effects like lowering of blood glucose etc, which give better chance to confirm therapeutic efficacy of unknown (test) compound.

4. There should be maximum possibility that individual variations must be minimised / accounted for. That means the estimation of error particularly related to biological variations should be possible so as to enable minimising the same. Biological variation is one of biggest problem encountered during bioassays although error/s by experimenter/s also play important role. Application of statistical procedure can lead to identity of variation and if the observations are meticulously recorded and studied, it can also guide on source of variation. In short many factors can contribute to variation in results which can be categorised as

    (a) *Biological factors:* Due the variations produced by experimental animal or its tissue, cell etc. The reasons can be – improper selection of animals i.e. some species and strains are known for either giving better or poor response in certain categories, variation in species; strain; age; sex of animal (may not always affect the outcome and sometimes it is advised to incorporate both sexes in the study) housing conditions including diet and timings of study. All these reasons for variations should be monitored.

    (b) *Experimenter factors:* Improper design of study by incorporating wrong animal species, selection of incorrect indicator (selected biological response to the drug) which either do not give enough (less sensitive), stable, sufficient and reproducible response to the given agent/ material and/ or sensitive to material other than subjected to test. The lack of required skill, errors in calculations of doses, dilutions, variations of experimental conditions (except animal) like change in materials, instrument; its sensitivity / magnifications etc.

(c) *Material Factors:* The material forms essential part of bioassay and includes everything except animals, may it be chemicals, glasswares, machines/instruments and balances etc. Any fault, error, quality problems in these materials can lead to giving undue variation in results.

The degree of pharmacological response produced should be reproducible under identical conditions [Eg Adrenaline shows same rise in BP in the same species under identical conditions: wt, age, sex, strain / breed etc]

5. Active principle to be assayed should show the same measured response in all animal species

6. Bioassay might measure a different aspect of the same substance compared to chemical assay [Eg testosterone & metabolites

Advantages and Disadvantages of Bioassays:

Advantages- They are important when- Chemical method is either not available or if available- it is too difficult due to complex nature and is less sensitive to detect the active constituent, Chemical composition or active principle of the given sample is not known or cannot be isolated in pure form and Chemical composition of drug differs but have the same pharmacological action and vice-versa, e.g. thyroid hormones etc.

Disadvantages: Bioassays, as compared to other methods of assays (e.g. chemical or physical assay) are less reproducible and less accurate at the same time they are expensive, time consuming and troublesome as compared to other (Physicochemical) methods. Further it demands more experimental skill of the performer. In addition, the factors affecting variations in results led to replacement of assay methods from bioassays to physicochemical / instrumental by most of the pharmacopoeias where ever it is possible. However, in case chemical assays and bioassays are giving contrasting outcomes, the result from bioassay should be considered as final because bioassay measure bioactive moieties present in given sample.

Methods of Bioassay: Although assays performed using cells, micro-organisms etc are also bioassays, conventionally the term bioassay is referred to the assays performed using animals and their tissues. Therefore the reported methods do not emphasize on methods relevant to cellular assays and mostly consist of methods for conducting assays on animals and their tissues. The given bioactive agent will produce certain response depending upon its nature. If it is agonist, it will produce positive response (change in given direction- whether increase or decrease) while antagonist will produce negative response (reduction in positive change produced with agonist). The response can be obtained in two ways- graded response or quantal response. Graded response means that the response is directly proportional to the dose and response will lie between no response and the maximum response as the dose increases till asymptote (i.e maximum response can be produced by the agent). The quantal response means that the response is reaching to a fixed quantity as envisaged by the experimenter. Therefore till that level is achieved, there is either no response or complete response. Thus it is in the form of "all or none", indicating that either it will reach to the target level (all) or it will not reach to target level (none). Simple example of this can be acute toxicity testing- either animal will die due to toxicity (all) or will not die (none) in given time. Third method is also there which is rarely used as bioassay but it involves measurement of response over a period of time (e.g. effect of vitamin in prevention / cure of disease over a period of time).

Considering that normally former two methods are applied, the bioassay can be conducted using any of the following type of Bioaasay-

1. ***Quantal or Direct End Point:*** In this type one has to set the endpoint of bioassay i.e any specific response to the given agent and the threshold dose producing a desired positive effect is measured on each animal. The comparison between the average results of two groups of animals (one receiving standard agent and other the test agent) is done. e.g. bioassay of insulin in mice. Two sets of experiment-one using standard insulin and the other using test or unknown insulin preparation are administered and by recording hypoglycaemic convulsion potency is calculated.

2. ***Interpolation:*** This is also called as Graphical Method as concentration of unknown is obtained from a standard plot of a log dose response curve of at least 4 sub maximal concentrations.

    This method is based on the principle of graded response making use of the dose-response relationship. Since dose – response curve is sigmoid curve, Log-dose vs response curve is plotted and the dose of standard producing the same response as produced by the test sample is interpolated from the graph. In the Graphical method of bioassay, the characteristic of log-dose response curve is linear in the middle (20-80%) portion of otherwise sigmoid dose- response curve. Therefore this range of doses of test and standard must be selected for getting better results. Usually one single response from one concentration of test drug suffices but if the situation permits more responses at different doses of test sample may be carried out. The concentration of test substance can be calculated by using calculation methods for Multiple Point assay (if more than one concentrations of test are administered) or interpolating the response from the graph plotted using standard drug concentrations.

Advantages: The method is a simple and better method. Particularly, if the test substance is scarce as only one point on standard graph suffices to lead for calculation of concentration of test. It also allows minimum errors as several responses of standard substances are taken and linearity is established between log dose and response.

3. *Matching :.* Initially two responses of the standard at different doses are taken in such a way that the response of one dose comes near lower end of dose response curve i. e. 20-25 % and second dose comes near higher end of DRC i.e near 70- 80 % of the maximum. The dose of test sample is kept constant to obtain single response lying between two responses of standard. After that different doses of standard are administered till equal responses to the test response are obtained. To confirm, the experiment is repeated with double dose of test and standard of which responses matched. If these are giving equal responses the appropriateness of the assay can be assumed and concentration of the test sample can be easily found out by comparing doses of test and standards as they are giving equal responses.

Advantages: It is easy as no calculations are involved and are of great utility where the sensitivity of the assay medium is varying as the test and standard are alternately given and at the end double doses are used.

Disadvantage: As many responses to be obtained, it is not suitable for test and standard agents that are costly or scarce at the same time consuming more time and paper for recording several responses. Other important constraint is the confirmation of matching the responses depend on perspective and skill of person and subjected to differences which can lead to error. Thus it is more laborious, less scientific and requires more amount of test and standard compounds.

4. *Bracketing Assays:* It is similar to above method except the response obtained by one dose of the test is bracketed by varying doses of standard till there is match is obtained between test dose and the standard dose. The order of responses can be started with lower dose of standard followed by test and higher dose of standard.

Multiple Point Assays

3 point assay: It combines principles of matching and interpolation by application of 2 doses of the standard and one dose of the test. Log dose response [LDR] curve plotted using response obtained from two varying concentration of standard solutions and given test solution. Select two standard doses s_1 & s_2 from linear part of LDR and the corresponding response be taken as S_1, S_2. A test dose t should be selected giving a corresponding response T, which will lie between S_1 & S_2. The experiment can be repeated with different order of sequence, i.e the Latin square method of randomization so as reduce error by avoiding bias, as follows-

- s_2 t s_1
- s_1 s_2 t
- s_2 s_1 t
- t s_1 s_2

4 point assay [combines principles of matching with interpolation]: In 4 point method 2 doses of standard and 2 doses of the test are used. In 6 point method 3 doses of standard and 3 doses of the test are used. Prepare log dose- response curve, select two standard doses s_1 & s_2 from linear part of it having corresponding response be S_1, S_2. Choose two test doses t_1 & t_2 with corresponding response T_1 & T_2 between S_1 & S_2. Usually the dose ratio of test and standard is kept at 2 i.e. $s_2/s_1 = t_2/t_1 = 2$.

Record 4 data sets [Latin square: Randomisation reduces error]

- t_1 t_2 s_1 s_2
- s_2 t_1 t_2 s_1
- t_2 s_1 s_2 t_1
- s_1 s_2 t_1 t_2

The mean of responses (S_1, S_2 and T_1, T_2) are obtained at corresponding doses.

Similarly assays with 6 Point, 8 Point etc are conducted to increase the precision of assays. E.g. 3 x 3 (6 Point) or 4 x4 (8 point) assay will enable to get two linear sets of data using log-dose vs. response curve. If both the lines are parallel, it indicates similarity between two groups i.e. test and standard. However, if the linearity is absent it indicates that there is either difference in active compounds, their combinations (if mixtures are present) or some interfering compound is present. If linear, one can easily point out differences by finding distance between two parallel lines and their slopes.

Bioassay of Antagonists: It involves the measurement and comparison of negative response i.e. reduction in response obtained by standard antagonist and the test antagonist. Thus one can choose any method, from the methods mentioned above, for assessing the antagonistic activity of test material. Simply in case of quantal assays- The changes in the quantal activity brought by standard antagonist and the test can be calculated. e. g. acute toxicity test of organophosphorus can be carried out by quantal response i e. quantum (number) of animal killed with given dose. If co-administration of suitable anticholinergic or enzyme activator can reduce the deaths, comparing reduction in deaths by administration of test agent and the standard can lead to calculation of potency or concentration of test. However, graded response methods are better suited for the bioassay of antagonist. Again any of the method i. e. graphical, multipoint, matching can be performed but interpolation / graphical method is more acceptable. The dose of agonist is fixed and the percentage inhibition of responses with different doses of test and standard antagonist are determined. Again the graph of log dose of antagonist and percent inhibition are plotted and the concentration of unknown can be determined by interpolation.

(The details with explaining practical examples and calculations are dealt in relevant sections in separate volumes of this book series by providing separate sections on different in-*vivo* and *in-vitro* experiments.)

10

Instrumentation in Experimental Pharmacology

Instrumentation plays important part in Experimental Pharmacology. It is highly important to know about equipments so as to extract better results and outcome of any study.

There are several instruments available for variety of purposes in Pharmacology experiments. Some are described here while others will be described in the experimental sections given in other volumes of this book series.

1. *Organ Bath Assembly:* This is group of simple instruments used for in-vitro tissue experiments. The details parts are shown in figure 10.1

   (i) *Perplex organ bath:* Made up of perplex (Polyacrylic) transparent material making it easy for observations. It have many openings either at side e.g. for heater and thermostat and at bottom i.e. for fitting organ tube and drainage of bath water. Tight sealing materials are used like rubber corks, gaskets etc to prevent leakage through the openings.

Sr. No.	Operations	Problems	Solving
1	Fill the bath with water	Leakages- a. From openings b. From sides/ bottom	a. Check gaskets / corks and fit it properly b. Rub the surfaces with cotton swab soaked in organic solvent like chloroform / ether etc if leakages are small. Apply adhesives like Araldite or Feviquick if leakage is large.
2	Make heater ON and check the temperature	No change in temperature	Get heater checked from electrician if everything is alright.

Contd...

Sr. No.	Operations	Problems	Solving
3	Set the temperature using thermostat- This needs patience. The setting has to be done slowly using 100^{0}C long thermometer (as it shows smaller graduations). Reset during different seasons. Fix the cellophane tape once the setting is confirmed (to avoid changes by mistake)	Temperature fluctuates from desired temp.	If the problem still persists refer it to the electrical expert. Note that it has only heater and if the room temp. goes above the desired (37^{0}C), switch off the heater and add cold water instead.

(ii) *Organ-tube:* The glass tube in which the tissue is placed during experiment as shown in the figure 10.1. It is available in several varieties of varying size and shape for different tissues. A silicon or rubber tube is attached at both openings at lower side- one for input of Physiological Salt solution and other for output. It is important to keep the output tube shorter by keeping pinch cock near glass organ tube to avoid over-dilution of drug present in the bath.

(iii) *Aeration tube:* cum- tissue holding unit- One end of this tube is attached to the tube linked to source of gas (either air through aerator or carbogen / oxygen from the cylinder) while other curved end is made suitable for tying one end of tissue. The small orifice allows the passage of gas in the perfusion fluid present in organ bath. It is firmly fitted with the clamp attached to metal stand fixed on the organ bath.

(iv) *Lever:* The suitable lever (Usually frontal writing) is attached to the stand fixed on Organ bath. It should be perpendicular to the plane of aeration tube to allow appropriate movements during responses. The thread tied to upper end of tissue is tied with lever in such a way that it will allow desired magnification of response. Before that lever must be balanced using suitable material like plasticine / mottling (china) clay to ensure that the lever will not produce strain on tissue due to the weight. The required load[1] can be adjusted during balancing so that it will not

---

[1] Load or Tension- It is the weight applied on tissue so as to relax the tissue after contractions due to drug effect. In some cases the load is continued through out the experiment to provide situation similar to body environment where tissue experiences tension due to adjoining organs/tissues. While in some cases load is removed during drug effect and again applied during relaxation to aid relaxation. (This problem was solved after communication- i.e Continuous footnote)

be done again. Otherwise weight is tied at equal distance from the fulcrum towards opposite side of tissue binding side.

(iv) *Kymograph:* It is mechanized unit allowing recording of responses on drum rotating at a variable speed (hence earlier machine was known as Sherrington Rotating Drum). It must be seen that while placing the drum and other operations the kymograph machine should be kept in neutral position otherwise the gears may get damaged. The speed can be set with speed selector, usually slow speed is selected for tissue contractions and high speed is selected for heart contractions or blood pressure measurement to balance the resolution in responses and prevent overuse of paper. The kymograph level must be balanced with help of screws provided at the bottom to prevent loss of accuracy due to either increased friction and impediment or losing the touch with paper leaving unrecorded response. Although it is not much affected with frontal writing lever as it has movable writing point, the responses with other levers like sideway writing lever, Starling heart lever can be greatly reduced due to imbalanced level of kymograph. The screw at the top of rotating axle enables adjustment of height of drum after it is placed on the knob for placing the drum and tightened the screw knob of drum. Before it the glazed paper (frictionless paper- to minimize reduction of response due to friction) is fixed on the drum in such a way that no glue is applied on drum to avoid roughening of its smooth surface and no wrinkles are present on paper. Now a days sketch pen tip is applied for recording response making the task of smoking obsolete. In older days the drum with paper wrapped around it was rotated on sooty flame produced by benzene + kerosene lamp. The experiments were to be conducted with utmost care as even smallest touch could spoil the smoked paper. After recording to preserve the tracings one had to fix the smoked paper by carefully dipping it in fixing solution like- wood coating solution (French polish), varnish, shellac or colophony solution (80-100 gm/ litre of organic solvent usually ethanol, methanol). The transparent layer formed over the tracing will not allow any change in to it – i.e. fixed.

(v) Aerator or Gas cylinder- The network of small plastic tubes is formed using small 4 way valves and T-s etc (usually used in small aquariums for aeration) in such a way that at every organ bath one aeration tube (tissue holder) is supplied one terminal for supply of gas/air. In this set up number of aerators can be reduced greatly (approximately $2/3^{rd}$ of total number of terminals. This can reduce expenditure on aerators and noise in laboratory due to too many aerators. If it is connected to gas cylinder it allows distribution of air to all the terminals in the laboratory. The air flow can be regulated by the flow regulators (valves) placed intermittently so that adequate gas is bubbled through the fluid. This not only provides the oxygen for tissue respiration but also stir the bath fluid causing better mixing of drug in all parts of fluid. The gas flow regulation is also important feature as less gas will not serve the purpose adequately and more bubbling with gas may lead to oxidation of tissue apart from turbulences in the tissue responses.

(vi) The reservoir – which supplies the fresh PSS to the organ bath through the glass coil attached to the side arm.

In Case of Power Failure: During experimentation power failure is not uncommon. There are 3 problems encountered due to sudden power failure-

(a) *Organ bath temperature maintenance:* This can be solved by placing thermometer in bath and adjusting it manually with warm water heated out side using water bath.

(b) *Stoppage of aerator:* This stops aeration and increases chances of death of tissue. It can be solved by pumping air with pipettes fitted with rubber bulb. The large scale solution to provide air can be use of small mechanical aerator (used by small goldsmiths or small tea makers for aeration of burning coal) and fitting it to the tube network. However if other gases are supplied using gas cylinder then no problem will arise due to power failure and will alleviate any measures to be taken.

(c) *Stopping of recording drum:* As mentioned above the speed is essential only in recording of rapid responses like measurement of heart rate or rapid twitches. Even the kymograph drum which is not rotating will enable to record the height of response. The drum should be kept in neutral position (See figure 10.1 showing neutral position of drum) and rotate the freely moving drum manually. It is must to rotate drum in neutral position as rotation of drum in geared position can damage the gears of the kymograph.

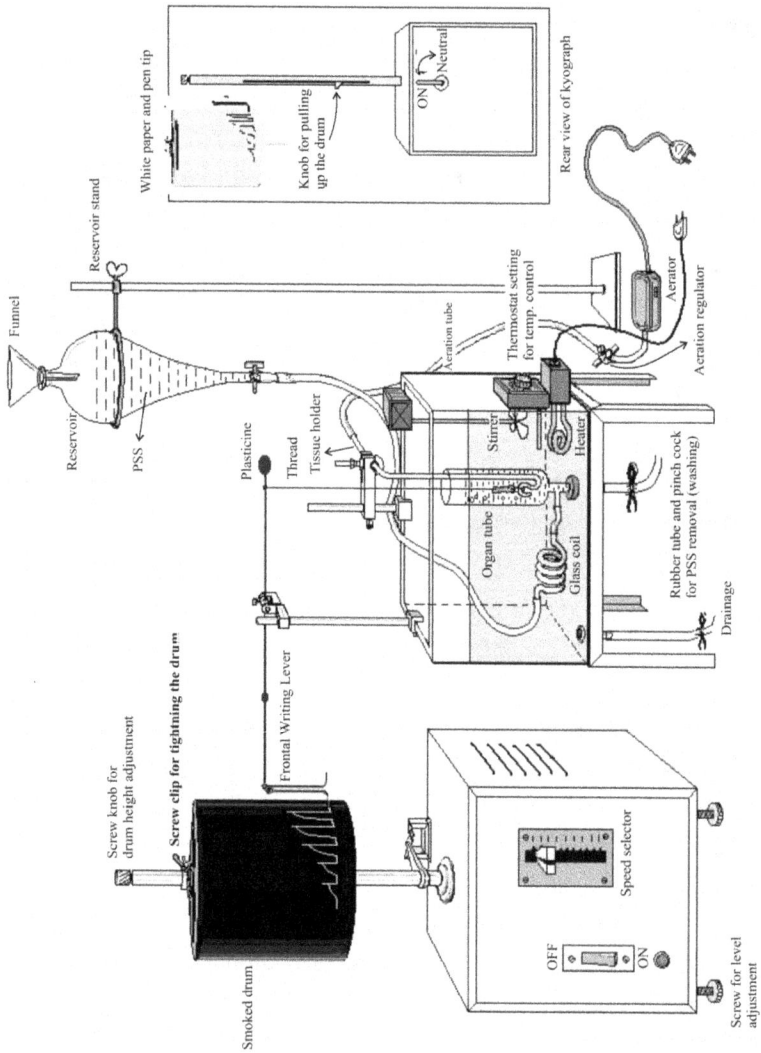

KYMOGRAPH   STUDENT'S ORGAN BATH ASSEMBLY

Figure 10.1 Assembly showing arrangement of organ bath, lever and kymograph

2. *Levers:* A lever is a simple machine that consists of a rigid bar supported at one point, known as the fulcrum. A force called the effort force is applied at one point on the lever in order to move an object, known as the resistance force, located at some other point on the lever. These are simple machines consisting of fulcrum allowing movement of the arms enabling to transmit the response. There are several types of levers used for transmitting the response to recorder instrument and acts as either first class (Fulcrum between effector and recording e.g. frontal, sideways etc) or second class levers (Fulcrum lies at one side and the effector and response lies at other side e.g. Starling, Brodies etc). There are 2 major types of levers- a. Isotonic and b. Isometric. a. Isotonic type- i.e. change in length due to contraction is recorded while the tension on the muscle remains the same e.g. simple lever frontal writing lever. (b) Isometric type-These levers are used under special circumstances for instance, when a twitch is produced by stimulating a muscle suspended between two rigid points, one being a strong spring, the muscle does not shorten but only creates a force or tension which is recorded; the twitch is also much faster in action.

Different types of lever

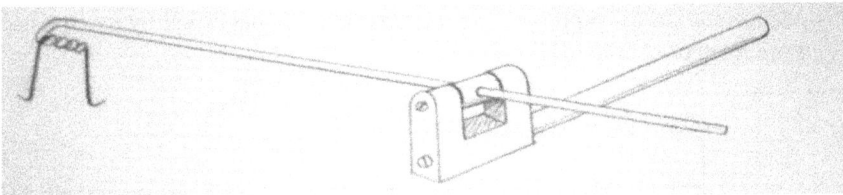

Frontal Writing lever

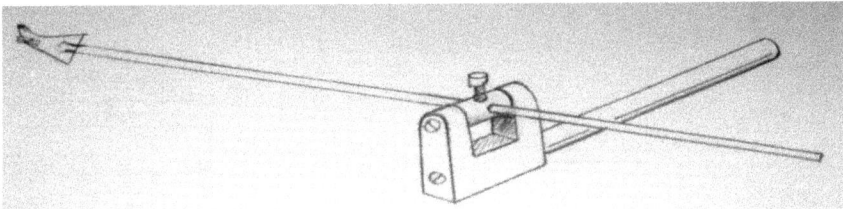

Sideways Writing Lever

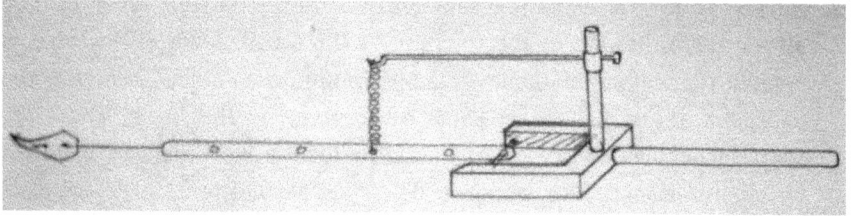

Starling Heart Lever

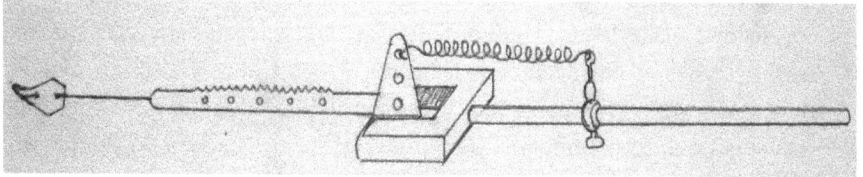

Brodie's lever

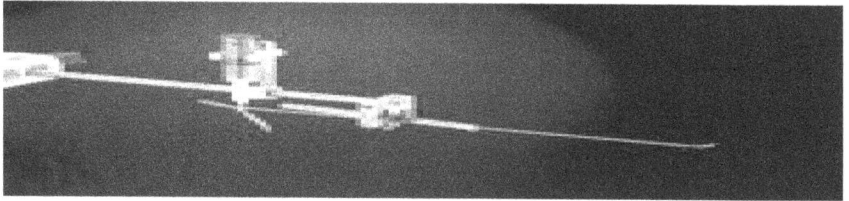

Gimbal Lever

Magnification of response- The response can be magnified by using basic principles of simple machines i.e.

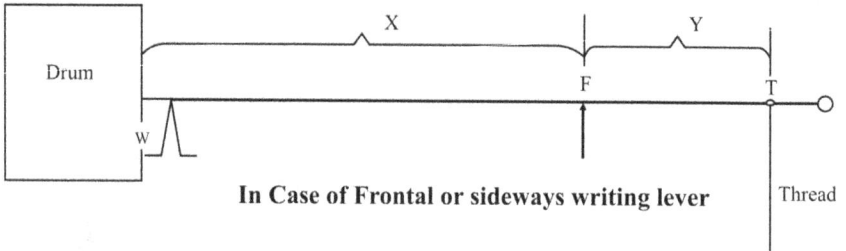

In Case of Frontal or sideways writing lever   Thread

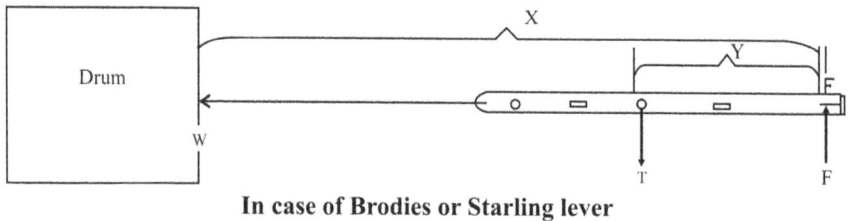

In case of Brodies or Starling lever

Where W- Writing point on recorder, F- The centre of Fulcrum, T- Point of attachment of tissue on lever.

The amount of magnification can be calculated as per equation given below-

Magnification of Response =

$$\frac{X}{Y} = \frac{\text{Distance between writing point (W) and Fulcrum (F)}}{\text{Distance between point of tissue attachment on lever (T) and Fulcrum}}$$

3. *Student Physiograph:* It is sophisticated recording unit giving several options for variety of experiments. They are more accurate, sensitive and give more resolution than the simple kymograph assembly which made them more acceptable for the research and most of the journals accept data only if the experiments are performed using such instruments. Their working is based on simple fact that the response input is converted in to electrical signals which are suitably amplified and converted in to mechanical output as observed on the recorders. Most important thing is single machine can be used for recording of multiple types of responses by changing components known as Transducers and Couplers. These instruments are also available as multiple units in single set and are called as polygraphs which are available as two to four channel physiographs. These allow simultaneous recording of more than one type of parameters with single machine. The polygraphs are useful when simultaneously more than one parameter is to be recorded. However while recording of single parameter it causes wastage of paper. Here the figure is displayed to show the 3- Channel Physiograph that will allow simultaneous recording of 3 parameters.

The physiograph can be divided in 3 parts which can be separated with each other-

1. *Main Unit:* The main unit can be divided in sections for better understanding- The front panel involving paper drive on-off switch, indicator light, buttons and knob for selecting paper speed and knob to lift pens along with window for paper feed. The top view shows the consol with many switches, knobs, sockets for variety of purposes. The big socket is provided for placing required coupler in which another socket is there for connecting transducer. The switches allows making mains on and off and Filter on-off while knobs are meant for selecting proper sensitivity, baseline and balance for acquiring data in most appropriate way as these allows setting response in particular range as envisaged by the experimenter.

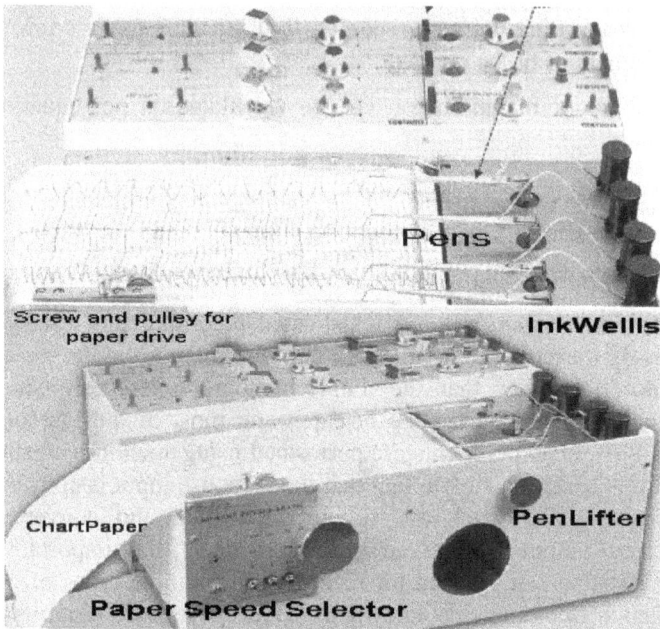

Screw and pulley for paper drive

Pens

InkWellls

ChartPaper

PenLifter

Paper Speed Selector

2. *Coupler:* The Unit which couples with appropriate transducer are called as Couplers. Various types of couplers are available for recording of different type of parameters and they should be used specifically with required transducer. Couplers should be housed in space provided inserting coupler in the consol. These provide the translation of signals received from transducer which converted in to mechanical output to move the pens. The coupler coupled with different transducer is mentioned in transducer section.

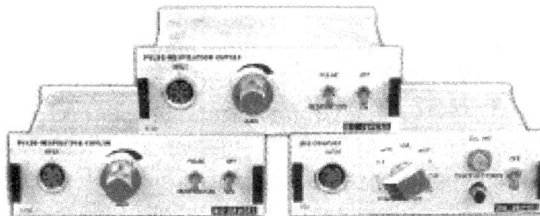

3. *Transducer:* This unit which transduces the response signals into electrical signals which are converted in to mechanical output by coupler and main unit. These are categorised below as per coupler required for it.

Since coupler and transducer are complementary to each other they are described together.

1. *Strain-Gauge Coupler:* This is coupled with the following transducers for the functions described below-

1		Pressure Transducer – This is used for measurement of pressure usually invasive blood pressure.
2		Respiration belt Transducer – This is modification of above which allows measurement of respiration rate.
3		Force Transducer – This usually are Isometric Force transducer which used for recording various contractions. Many variants with different load and displacement (as measured in terms of mass displaced unit- mg/gm etc)
4		Volume Transducer – this can be used for measurement of volume like, plethysmography i.e. inflammation measurement etc.

2. *Pulse-Respiration and NIBP Coupler:*

5		Respiration Transducer – can be used for measurement of various respiratory parameters
6		Pulse Transducer – Measures pulse rate

3. *Temperature Coupler:* This is coupled with temperature transducer.

7		Temperature Transducer- Measurement of temperature as explained in telethermometer.

4. *Isotonic Coupler:* Some physiograph manufacturers provides separate coupler for isotonic transducer while in some cases it may not exist as the transducer can be attached with SGC

8		Isotonic Transducer – For recording contraction of smooth muscles like aorta requiring very sensitive recording system.

5. *Biopotential Coupler:* This coupler is used for recording the changes in potential during various functions like ElectroCardiogram (ECG) is used for recording changes in potential during cardiac cycle, ElectroMyogram (EMG) is used for recording changes in muscle potential during contractions and relaxations, Electro Encephalogram (EEG) is used for measurement of potential in brain. The slight modification of the same is

	provided by some physiograph manufacturers as an electrocardiogram coupler for recording human ECG only with setting for selecting different leads	
9		3 PIN/ 5 PIN Junction Box - Are used to connect the electrodes for measurement of various potential.

After assembling the instrument set the baseline, sensitivity and balance for getting best mix of sensitivity and resolution of the response by adjusting the minimum and maximum response. It is must to refer the Operation manual as different manufacturer suggest slight variation in the operation. It is also must to get the instrument calibrated before starting the actual animal or human experiment. This not only assures standardised responses but also give information about mechanical functioning of instrument as many a times if the instrument is used after long gap the chances of clogging of writer pens due to packing the instrument without cleaning the pen either after removal of ink or without removing ink. The trial also verifies the paper movement. Thus it is necessary to take care of instrument after finishing work by carefully cleaning it and keeping all the delicate parts carefully in cupboard or such closed box not allowing dust or rodents to ruin it.

4. *Advanced Physiographs:* Fortunately, the author could experience the tremendous benefits offered by advanced system like Biopac four channel Physiograph during his research. Many such advanced systems are available, commonly referred as **Data Acquisition Systems** like Biopac, Powerlab and many more. Although their basic functions are similar to that of student Physiograph, these systems differs on many counts- they are more sensitive, more accurate, give better resolution due to support of highly developed softwares compatible with their instruments and giving several computational expansions of the acquired data using many algorithms in the software. These systems must be attached to a computer for acquiring the data using the software provided by the supplier. This data is stored in computer and can be used as and when required. This format allows many treatments like magnification, rate of recording, maximising view of only one or more channels without affecting recording through other channels. Given below is example of recording we have obtained using Biopac data acquisition system during our research on myocardial ischemia- reperfusion injury.

The system enabled us to record blood pressure, ECG and temperature simultaneously. From these recording the software automatically gives dp/dt an important parameter for cardiovascular studies, details of specific parameters of ECG like R-amplitude. ST-elongation and ST-elevation, heart rate etc.. In short such highly sophisticated instruments enables to have more details about the parameters which lead to better conclusions.

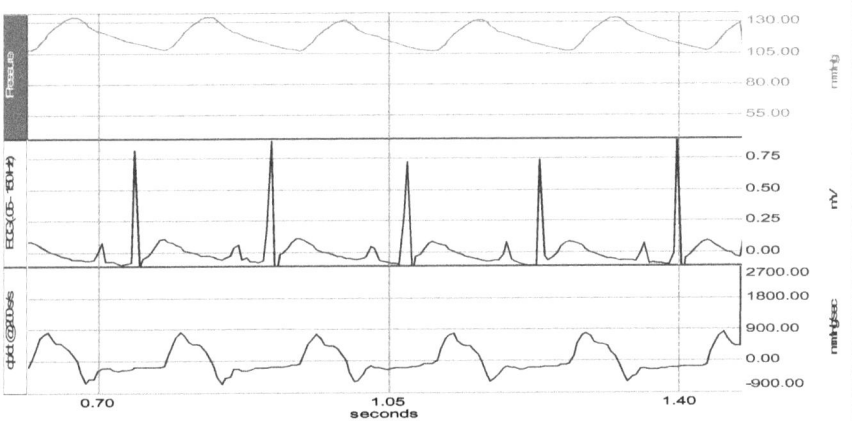

Showing blood pressure (top), ECG (middle) and dp/dt (bottom) of control animals.

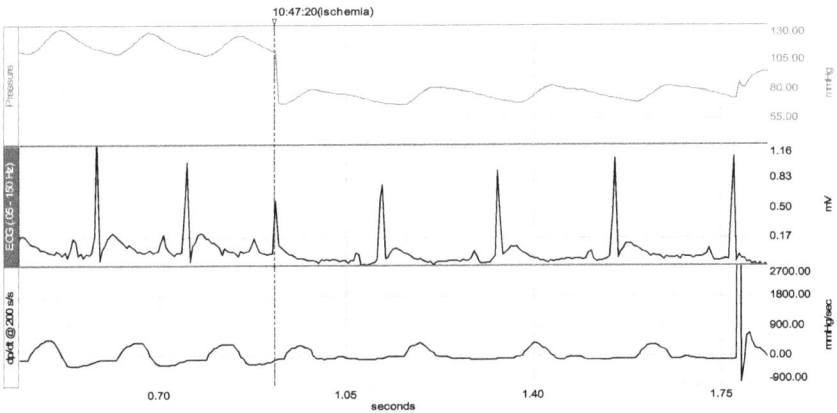

Showing changes in blood pressure (top), ECG (middle) and dp/dt (bottom) of control animals at the time of ischemia

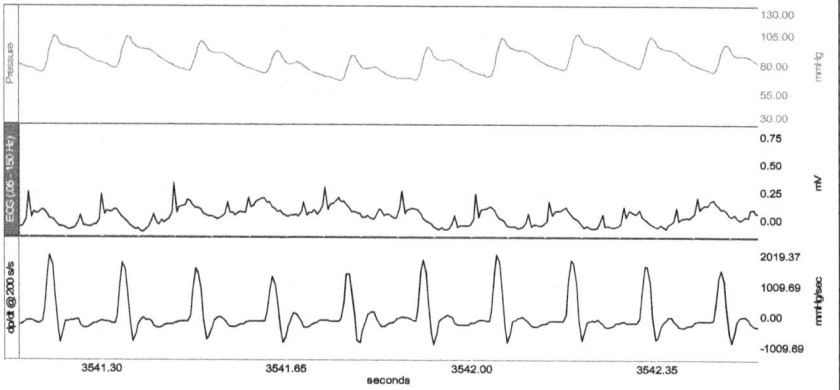

Showing changes in blood pressure (top), ECG (middle) and dp/dt (bottom) of control animals at the time of ischemia

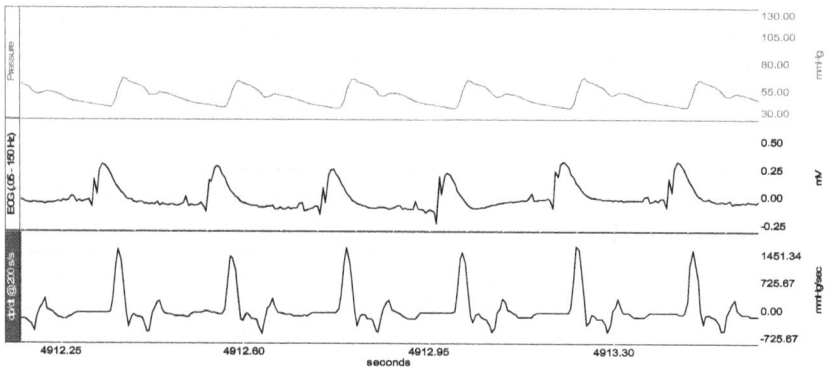

Showing changes in blood pressure (top), ECG (middle) and dp/dt (bottom) of control animals at the time of ischemia

Other Common laboratory equipments: Many other instruments are used in Pharmacology and their detailed use will be described in coming sections. However brief introduction is hereby given for information.

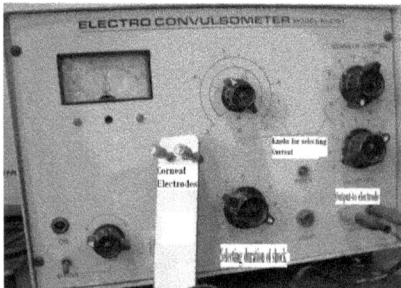

Electro convulsiometer: This instrument is used to study anti-convulsant activity using electrically induced convulsions in animals using either ear lobe electrodes or corneal electrode (as shown in figure). The instrument allows selecting appropriate current for desired duration by rotating knobs provided for various functions.

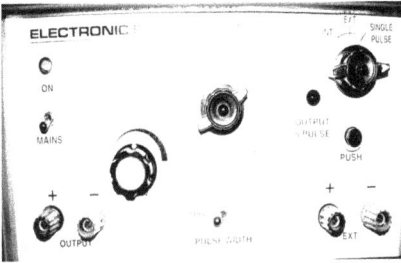

Stimulator- This instrument is used to apply required amount of current to tissue using different electrode. The instrument allows selecting appropriate current and whether in single or in pulsatile way for desired duration by rotating knobs provided for various functions. This instrument is used for study of physiology and effects of drug at neuromuscular junction.

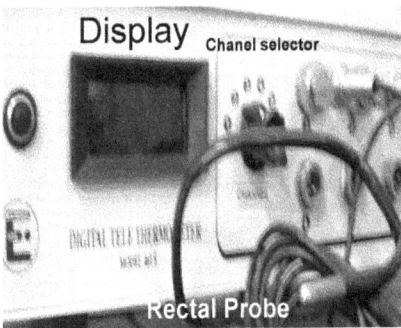

Digital Telethermometer- This instrument is used to study changes in temperature in animal body by inserting rectal probes. This can be used for studying antipyretic effect, noting the changes in body temperature due to various reasons, pyrogen assays etc. The input from rectal probes reaches to consol and converted in to digital signals showing temperature on display. The instrument should be calibrated by dipping probe in to water with known temperature.

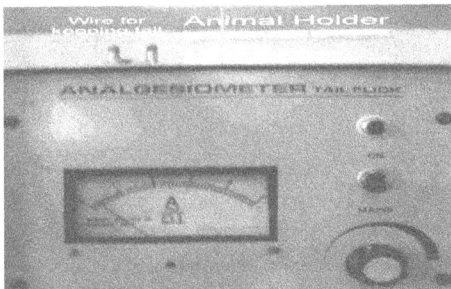

Analgesiometer

(Tail Flick): This instrument is used to study effect of analgesics on rat by keeping it in animal holder and placing tail on hot wire to observe the time taken for flicking the tail. Analgesic will increase the pain threshold thereby increasing the time required to flick the tail.

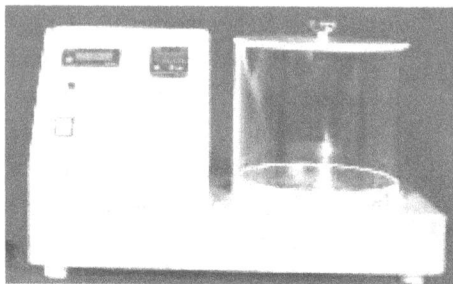

Analgesiometer (Hot Plate): This instrument is used to study effect of analgesics on rat by keeping it on hot plate to observe the time taken for licking the paws or showing such signs. Analgesic will increase the pain threshold thereby increasing the time required to lick the paw.

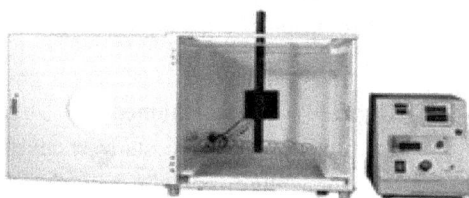

Pole Climbing Apparatus: the instrument provides tool for screening antipsychotic drugs using various modes to observe effects on conditioned response.

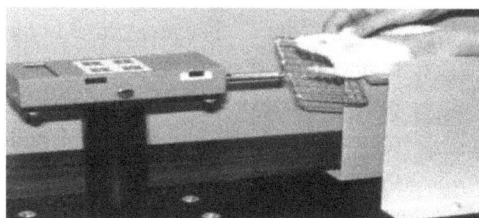

Grip Strength Tester: The instrument is used for assessment of drugs acting on neuromuscular junction, muscular system and CNS. It will measure force

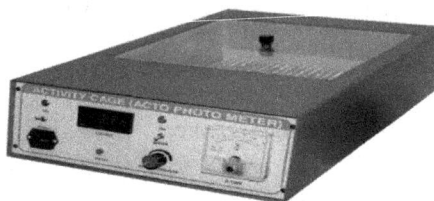

Actophotometer: Also known as activity cage, allows measurement of spontaneous activity and effect of various agents acting on CNS on the spontaneous activity.

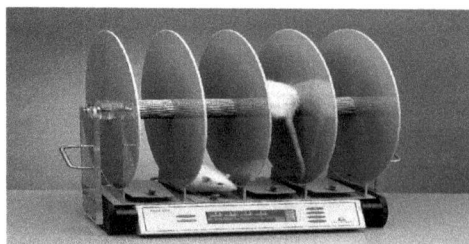

Rota Rod: The instrument is used for assessment of drugs acting on neuromuscular junction, muscular system and CNS.

There are many other instruments that can be used in experimental Pharmacology. Here only those instruments used frequently during undergraduate pharmacology experiments are explained. Several instruments might be essential for pharmacologists while assessing the activities using various models and parameters. The range is very broad and some these are briefly discussed below-

CNS Studies: Stereotaxic apparatus for locating specific area in brain enabling either placing electrodes for EEG or micro drill for administration at particular area of brain. Various mazes- plus maze, Y- maze, 8-maze etc, hole board and many more to explore behavioural changes in animals with respect to induction of disease or effect of treatment.

Cardiovascular Studies: Apart from highly sensitive transducers as explained above many other instruments / techniques are available for the cardiovascular recording e.g. Non-invasive blood pressure (NIBP), Telemetry – The sensors sensing blood pressure, ECG are placed in animals and the recordings can be done during their normal locomotor activities in the cage. This gives more true information negating the effect of anaesthesia and surgery.

Analytical: Ranging from bioanalytical to purely analytical instruments are used e.g. auto analyser for various biochemical parameters in biological fluids, microplate readers for its versatility in applications, spectrophotometers, HPLC etc.

Biotechnology – Several instruments and related techniques like electrophoresis, pCR, cell isolation, DNA/ RNA/ Protein isolation and quantification are some the instrumental techniques that are used during research activities in Pharmacology.

In addition other diagnostic tools like X- ray, MRI, endoscopy, histopathological studies etc can also be used to confirm many parameters of the study.

The combination of such advanced instruments and technology is used for rapid Pharmacological screening of agents to enable fast out come. The technique is known as High Throughput Screening (HTS) which employ many techniques of biotechnology, analytical and data acquisition to yield information regarding the activity of given entity. This technique is very fast and thousands of compounds per day can be studied with the instrument. The receptors / enzymes obtained using biotechnology are placed in wells of microplates and suitable mechanism to identify the changes in these biological moieties due to addition of agents capable to make the changes are devised. The detectors to quantify such changes are placed in instrument.

The detectors are usually based on analytical techniques like absorption of light using spectrophotometric / fluorescence / phosphorescence or other such technique or combination of such techniques, enabling detection in the outcome due to combination of drug and biological moiety. The computerised data acquisition system collects and collates data to give information. The compounds with slight activity are separated as Hits, with moderate activity are selected as Leads and the compounds with better activity with safer margin are converted in to New Chemical Entity (NCE). The hits and leads can be structurally modified using structure activity relation ship studies to get optimization i.e. more activity and fewer adverse effects.

11

Data Analyses and Use of Computers

The application of statistics starts with randomization of subjects /animals available for study to minimize errors, bias etc leading to failure of study and it ends with final data analysis confirming whether the results are acceptable or not. Suppose that data from two samples of animals treated with different drugs is collected in which an enzyme in each animal's plasma is measured and the means are different. It will be essential to know whether that difference is due to an effect of the drug – whether the two populations have different means. Observing different sample means is not enough to persuade anyone to conclude that the populations have different means. It is possible that the populations have the same mean (i.e., that the drugs have no effect on the enzyme you are measuring) and that the difference observed between sample means occurred only by chance. There is no way one can ever be sure if the observed difference reflects a true difference or if it simply occurred in the course of random sampling. All one can do is calculate probabilities.

Statistical calculations can answer this question: In an experiment of this size, if the populations really have the same mean, what is the probability of observing at least as large a difference between sample means as was, in fact, observed? The answer to this question is called the *P value*.

The P value is a probability, with a value ranging from zero to one. If the P value is small enough, it can be concluded that the difference between sample means is unlikely to be due to chance indicating that the populations have different means.

What is a null hypothesis?

When statisticians discuss P values, they use the term *null hypothesis*. The null hypothesis simply states that there is no difference between the groups. Using that term, you can define the P value to be the probability of observing a difference as large as or larger than you observed if the null hypothesis were true.

Common misinterpretation of a P value

Many people misunderstand P values. If the P value is 0.05, it means that there is a 5% chance of observing a difference as large as one has observed even if the two population means are identical (the null hypothesis is true). It is tempting to conclude, therefore, that there is a 95% chance that the difference you observed reflects a real difference between populations and a 5% chance that the difference is due to chance. However, this would be an incorrect conclusion. What you can say is that random sampling from identical populations would lead to a difference smaller than you observed in 97% of experiments and larger than you observed in 5% of experiments. One-tail vs. two-tail P values-

When comparing two groups, you must distinguish between one- and two-tail P values. Both one- and two-tail P values are based on the same null hypothesis, that two populations really are the same and that an observed discrepancy between sample means is due to chance.

Definition of power: Start with the assumption that two population means differ by a certain amount, but have the same SD. Now assume that we have to perform many experiments with the appropriate sample size, and calculate a P value for each experiment. Power is the fraction of these experiments that would lead to statistically significant results, i.e., would have a P value less than alpha (the largest P value you deem "significant", usually set to 0.05). In short, it gives idea about minimum subjects/ animals to be used to get statistical significant results. This can be better understood using CAL simulation explained in chapter 4 (III. 4- sample size and power calculation)

Paired or unpaired test?

When choosing a test, one has to decide whether to use a paired test. A paired test can be chosen when the two columns of data are matched. Here are some examples:

- measure a variable (e.g., weight) before an intervention, and then measure it in the same subjects after the intervention.
- recruit subjects as pairs, matched for variables such as age, ethnic group, and disease severity. One of the pair gets one treatment; the other gets an alternative treatment.

- run a laboratory experiment several times, each time with a control and treated preparation handled in parallel.
- measure a variable in twins or child/parent pairs.

More generally, one should select a paired test whenever it is expected that a value in one group to be closer to a *particular* value in the other group than to a *randomly selected* value in the other group.

Computers have almost replaced manual methods for numerical calculations in Experimental Pharmacology. These are not only accurate but also very fast to perform and reduce considerable amount of time.

Brief introduction of various statistical functions is given in next sections of this chapter. Since manual calculations are not expected, equations are not given in the text and attempts are made to explain how to use software for some important tasks during Pharmacology Experiments. Many softwares are available for statistical application in Biological Sciences i.e Biostatistics. Some of these are- Graphpad prizm, SSPS, systat etc. All these are having several tools and can satisfy most of the needs of the experimenters. However the cost is quite high. At the same time Microsoft Excel can also perform several tasks and easily available. The effort is made to explain the applications available with Excel that can be used for data analysis during Pharmacology experiments.

Statistical analysis tools

Microsoft Excel provides a set of data analysis tools— called the Analysis ToolPak— that can be used to save steps when one develop complex statistical or engineering analyses. One provides the data and parameters for each analysis; the tool uses the appropriate statistical or engineering macro functions and then displays the results in an output table. Some tools generate charts in addition to output tables.

Related worksheet functions Excel provides many other statistical, financial, and engineering worksheet functions. Some of the statistical functions are built-in and others become available when the Analysis ToolPak is installed.

Accessing the data analysis tools The Analysis ToolPak includes the tools described below. To access these tools, click **Data Analysis** on the **Tools** menu. If the **Data Analysis** command is not available, one need to load the Analysis ToolPak add-in program.

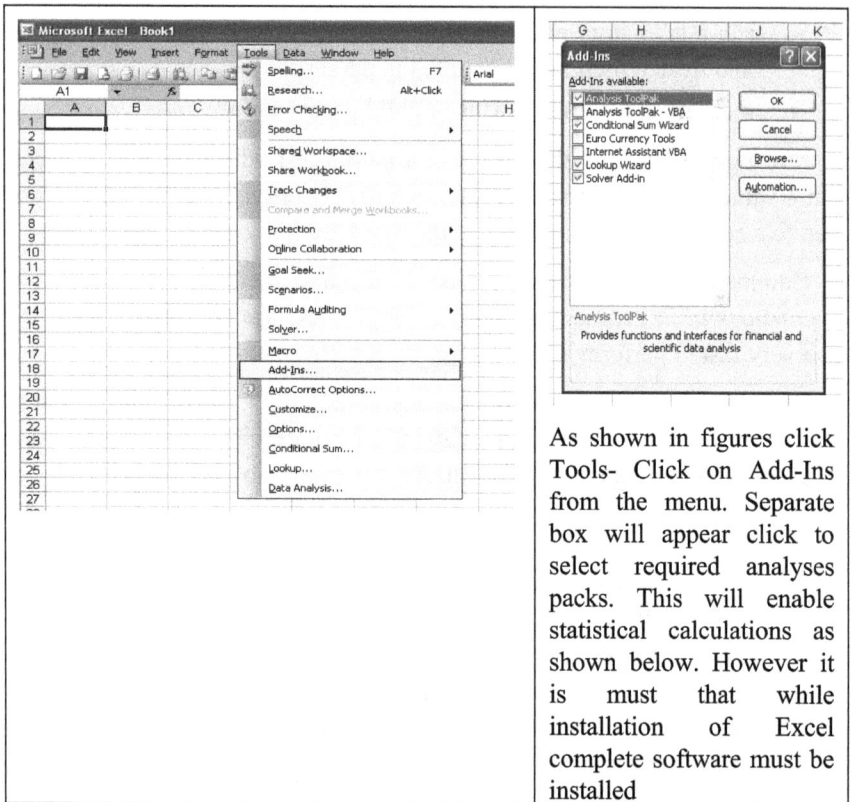

As shown in figures click Tools- Click on Add-Ins from the menu. Separate box will appear click to select required analyses packs. This will enable statistical calculations as shown below. However it is must that while installation of Excel complete software must be installed

ANOVA-The Anova analysis tools provide different types of variance analysis. The tool to use depends on the number of factors and the number of samples one have from the populations to be tested.

Anova: **Single Factor** This tool performs a simple analysis of variance on data for two or more samples. The analysis provides a test of the hypothesis that each sample is drawn from the same underlying probability distribution against the alternative hypothesis that underlying probability distributions are not the same for all samples. If there were only two samples, the worksheet function, TTEST, could equally well be used. With more than two samples, there is no convenient generalization of TTEST and the Single Factor Anova model should be used.

One-way ANOVA (and related nonparametric tests) compare three or more groups when the data are categorized in one way. For example, one might compare a control group with two treated groups. After application of ANOVA if some one wishes to confirm differences at inter-group level can apply post test. Choosing an appropriate post test is not easy as different statistics texts make different recommendations. The application of post test is possible with the use of biostatistics softwares mentioned above.

Select **Dunnett's** test if one column represents control data and all other columns are to be compared with control column but not to each other.

Select the **test for linear trend** if the columns are arranged in a natural order (e.g. dose or time) and one wants to test whether there is a trend such that values increase (or decrease) as experimenter moves from left to right across columns.

Select the **Bonferroni test for selected pairs of columns** when certain column pairs are to be compared. Select those pairs based on experimental design and ideally should specify the pairs of interest before collecting any data.

If you want to compare all pairs of columns, you have three choices: the Bonferroni, Tukey, or Newman-Keuls (also known as the Student-Newman-Keuls or SNK) tests. The only advantage of the Bonferroni method is that it is easy to understand. Its disadvantage is that it is too conservative, so you are more apt to miss real differences (also confidence intervals are too wide). This is a minor concern when you compare only a few columns, but is a major problem when you have many columns. Don't use the Bonferroni test with more than five groups. Choosing between the **Tukey** and **Newman-Keuls** test is not straightforward, and there appears to be no real consensus among statisticians. The two methods are related, and the rationale for the differences is subtle. The methods are identical when comparing the largest group mean with the smallest. For other comparisons, the Newman-Keuls test yields lower P values. The problem is that it is difficult to articulate exactly what null hypotheses the Newman-Keuls P values test. For that reason, and because the Newman-Keuls test does not generate confidence intervals, we suggest selecting Tukey's test. (If you select the Tukey test, you are actually selecting the Tukey-Kramer test, which includes the extension by Kramer to allow for unequal sample sizes.)

Anova: **Two-Factor With Replication** This analysis tool is useful when data can be classified along two different dimensions. For example, in an experiment to measure the effect of various drugs (for example, X, Y, Z) on blood pressure, and also effect of diet (for example, low, high salt). For each of the 6 possible pairs of {drugs, diet} we have an equal number of observations of blood pressure. Using this Anova tool we can test:

1. Whether blood pressures of the subjects using different drugs are drawn from the same underlying population; dietary conditions are ignored for this analysis.

2. Whether blood pressures of the subjects using different dietary conditions are drawn from the same underlying population; fertilizer brands are ignored for this analysis.

3. Whether having accounted for the effects of differences between effects of drugs found in step 1 and differences in dietary conditions found in step 2, the 6 samples representing all pairs of {drugs, dietary condition} values are drawn from the same population. The alternative hypothesis is that there are effects due to specific { drugs, dietary condition } pairs over and above differences based on drug alone or on diet alone.

Thus it can be used for answering some questions: 1. Does the first factor systematically affect the results? In our example: Are the mean responses the same for all three drugs? 2. Does the second factor systematically affect the results? In our example: Are the mean responses the same for drugs and dietary conditions? 3. Do the two factors interact? Although the outcome measure (dependent variable) is a continuous variable, each factor must be categorical.

Anova: **Two-Factor Without Replication** This analysis tool is useful when data are classified on two different dimensions as in the Two-Factor case With Replication. However, for this tool we assume that there is only a single observation for each pair (for example, each { drugs, dietary condition } pair in the example above. Using this tool we can apply the tests in steps 1 and 2 of the Anova: Two-Factor With Replication case but do not have enough data to apply the test in step 3.

Correlation

The CORREL and PEARSON worksheet functions both calculate the correlation coefficient between two measurement variables when measurements on each variable are observed for each of N subjects. (Any missing observation for any subject causes that subject to be ignored in the analysis.) The Correlation analysis tool is particularly useful when there are more than two measurement variables for each of N subjects. It provides an output table, a correlation matrix, showing the value of CORREL (or PEARSON) applied to each possible pair of measurement variables.

The correlation coefficient, like the covariance, is a measure of the extent to which two measurement variables "vary together." Unlike the covariance, the correlation coefficient is scaled so that its value is independent of the units in which the two measurement variables are expressed. (For example, if the two measurement variables are weight and height, the value of the correlation coefficient is unchanged if weight is converted from pounds to kilograms.) The value of any correlation coefficient must be between -1 and +1 inclusive.

One can use the correlation analysis tool to examine each pair of measurement variables to determine whether the two measurement variables tend to move together— that is, whether large values of one variable tend to be associated with large values of the other (positive correlation), whether small values of one variable tend to be associated with large values of the other (negative correlation), or whether values of both variables tend to be unrelated (correlation near zero).

Covariance

The Correlation and Covariance tools can both be used in the same setting, when one have N different measurement variables observed on a set of individuals. The Correlation and Covariance tools each give an output table, a matrix, showing the correlation coefficient or covariance, respectively, between each pair of measurement variables. The difference is that correlation coefficients are scaled to lie between -1 and +1 inclusive, Corresponding covariances are not scaled. Both the correlation coefficient and the covariance are measures of the extent to which two variables "vary together."

The Covariance tool computes the value of the worksheet function, COVAR, for each pair of measurement variables. (Direct use of COVAR rather than the Covariance tool is a reasonable alternative when there are only two measurement variables, i.e. N=2.) The entry on the diagonal of the Covariance tool's output table in row i, column i is the covariance of the i-th measurement variable with itself; this is just the population variance for that variable as calculated by the worksheet function, VARP.

One can use the covariance tool to examine each pair of measurement variables to determine whether the two measurement variables tend to move together— that is, whether large values of one variable tend to be associated with large values of the other (positive covariance), whether small values of one variable tend to be associated with large values of the other (negative covariance), or whether values of both variables tend to be unrelated (covariance near zero).

Descriptive Statistics

The Descriptive Statistics analysis tool generates a report of univariate statistics for data in the input range, providing information about the central tendency and variability of the data.

Exponential Smoothing

The Exponential Smoothing analysis tool predicts a value based on the forecast for the prior period, adjusted for the error in that prior forecast. The tool uses the smoothing constant a, the magnitude of which determines how strongly forecasts respond to errors in the prior forecast.

Note: Values of 0.2 to 0.3 are reasonable smoothing constants. These values indicate that the current forecast should be adjusted 20 to 30 percent for error in the prior forecast. Larger constants yield a faster response but can produce erratic projections. Smaller constants can result in long lags for forecast values.

F-Test Two-Sample for Variances

The F-Test Two-Sample for Variances analysis tool performs a two-sample F-test to compare two population variances.

For example, one can use the F-test tool on samples of times in a swim meet for each of two teams. The tool provides the result of a test of the null hypothesis that these two samples come from distributions with equal variances against the alternative that the variances are not equal in the underlying distributions.

The tool calculates the value f of an F-statistic (or F-ratio). A value of f close to 1 provides evidence that the underlying population variances are equal. In the output table, if f < 1 "P(F <= f) one-tail" gives the probability of observing a value of the F-statistic less than f when population variances are equal and "F Critical one-tail" gives the critical value less than 1 for the chosen significance level, Alpha. If f > 1, "P(F <= f) one-tail" gives the probability of observing a value of the F-statistic greater than f when population variances are equal and "F Critical one-tail" gives the critical value greater than 1 for Alpha.

Fourier Analysis

The Fourier Analysis tool solves problems in linear systems and analyzes periodic data by using the Fast Fourier Transform (FFT) method to transform data. This tool also supports inverse transformations, in which the inverse of transformed data returns the original data.

Histogram

The Histogram analysis tool calculates individual and cumulative frequencies for a cell range of data and data bins. This tool generates data for the number of occurrences of a value in a data set.

For example, in a class of 20 students, one could determine the distribution of scores in letter-grade categories. A histogram table presents the letter-grade boundaries and the number of scores between the lowest bound and the current bound. The single most-frequent score is the mode of the data.

Moving Average

The Moving Average analysis tool projects values in the forecast period, based on the average value of the variable over a specific number of preceding periods. A moving average provides trend information that a simple average of all historical data would mask. Use this tool to forecast sales, inventory, or other trends.

Random Number Generation

The Random Number Generation analysis tool fills a range with independent random numbers drawn from one of several distributions. One can characterize subjects in a population with a probability distribution. For example, one might use a normal distribution to characterize the population of individuals' heights, or one might use a Bernoulli distribution of two possible outcomes to characterize the population of coin-flip results.

Rank and Percentile

The Rank and Percentile analysis tool produces a table that contains the ordinal and percentage rank of each value in a data set. One can analyze the relative standing of values in a data set. This tool uses the worksheet functions, RANK and PERCENTRANK. RANK does not account for tied values. If one wish to account for tied values, use the worksheet function, RANK, together with the correction factor suggested in the help file for RANK.

Regression

The Regression analysis tool performs linear regression analysis by using the "least squares" method to fit a line through a set of observations. One can analyze how a single dependent variable is affected by the values of one or more independent variables.

For example, one can analyze how an athlete's performance is affected by such factors as age, height, and weight. One can apportion shares in the performance measure to each of these three factors, based on a set of performance data, and then use the results to predict the performance of a new, untested athlete.

The Regression tool uses the worksheet function, LINEST.

Sampling

The Sampling analysis tool creates a sample from a population by treating the input range as a population. When the population is too large to process or chart, one can use a representative sample. One can also create a sample that contains only values from a particular part of a cycle if one believes that the input data is periodic.

For example, if the input range contains quarterly sales figures, sampling with a periodic rate of four places values from the same quarter in the output range.

t-Test -The Two-Sample t-Test analysis tools test for equality of the population means underlying each sample. The three tools employ different assumptions: that the population variances are equal, that the population variances are not equal, and that the two samples represent before treatment and after treatment observations on the same subjects.

For all three tools below, a t-Statistic value, t, is computed and shown as "t Stat" in the output tables. Depending on the data, this value, t, can be negative or non-negative. Under the assumption of equal underlying population means, if t < 0, "P(T <= t) one-tail" gives the probability that a value of the t-Statistic would be observed that is more negative than t. If t >=0, "P(T <= t) one-tail" gives the probability that a value of the t-Statistic would be observed that is more positive than t. "t Critical one-tail" gives the cutoff value so that the probability of observing a value of the t-Statistic greater than or equal to "t Critical one-tail" is Alpha.

"P(T <= t) two-tail" gives the probability that a value ot the t-Statistic would be observed that is larger in absolute value than t. "P Critical two-tail" gives the cutoff value so that the probability of an observed t-Statistic larger in absolute value than "P Critical two-tail" is Alpha.

t-Test: **Two-Sample Assuming Equal Variances** This analysis tool performs a two-sample student's t-test. This t-test form assumes that the two data sets came from distributions with the same variances. It is referred to as a homoscedastic t-test. One can use this t-test to determine whether the two samples are likely to have come from distributions with equal population means.

t-Test: **Two-Sample Assuming Unequal Variances** This analysis tool performs a two-sample student's t-test. This t-test form assumes that the two data sets came from distributions with unequal variances. It is referred to as a heteroscedastic t-test. As with the Equal Variances case above, one can use this t-test to determine whether the two samples are likely to have come from distributions with equal population means. Use this test when the there are distinct subjects in the two samples. Use the Paired test, described below,when there is a single set of subjects and the two samples represent measurements for each subject before and after a treatment.

t-Test: **Paired Two Sample For Means** One can use a paired test when there is a natural pairing of observations in the samples, such as when a sample group is tested twice— before and after an experiment. This analysis tool and its formula perform a paired two-sample student's t-test to determine whether observations taken before a treatment and observations taken after a treatment are likely to have come from distributions with equal population means. This t-test form does not assume that the variances of both populations are equal.

z-Test: The z-Test: Two Sample for Means analysis tool performs a two-sample z-test for means with known variances. This tool is used to test the null hypothesis that there is no difference between two population means against either one-sided or two-sided alternative hypotheses . If variances are not known, the worksheet function, ZTEST, should be used instead.

When using the z-Test tool, one should be careful to understand the output. "P(Z <= z) one-tail" is really P(Z >= ABS(z)), the probability of a z-value further from 0 in the same direction as the observed z value when there is no difference between the population means. "P(Z <= z) two-tail" is really P(Z >= ABS(z) or Z <= -ABS(z)), the probability of a z-value further from 0 in either direction than the observed z-value when there is no difference between the population means. The two-tailed result is just the one-tailed result multiplied by 2. The z-Test tool can also be used for the case where the null hypothesis is that there is a specific non-zero value for the difference between the two population means.

For example, one can use this test to determine differences between the performances of two car models

Use of Excel for some functions in experimental Pharmacology

I. Randomiztion

dialog box-

Number of Variables- Enter the number of columns of values in the output table as per need. If number is not entered, Excel will automatically fill all columns in the output range as specified.

Number of Random Numbers- Enter the number of data points as desired. Each data point appears in a row of the output table. If number is not entered, Excel will automatically fill all rows in the output range as specified.

Distribution- Click the distribution method from the following to use to create random values.

Uniform-Characterized by lower and upper bounds. Variables are drawn with equal probability from all values in the range. A common application uses a uniform distribution in the range 0...1.

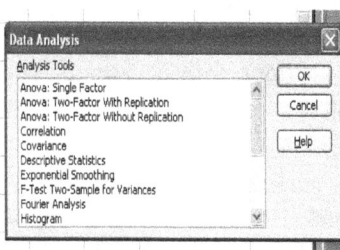

In the data analysis window the last tool in Analysis Tools box is Random Number Generation. Click the same and click OK. Apply it to the given data and select the choices as per the need. The details are given in neighbouring box.

Normal -Characterized by a mean and a standard deviation. A common application uses a mean of 0 and a standard deviation of 1 for the standard normal distribution.

Bernoulli-Characterized by a probability of success (p value) on a given trial. Bernoulli random variables have the value 0 or 1. For example, you can draw a uniform random variable in the range 0...1. If the variable is less than or equal to the probability of success, the Bernoulli random variable is assigned the value 1; otherwise, it is assigned the value 0.

Binomial-Characterized by a probability of success (p value) for a number of trials. For example, you can generate number-of-trials Bernoulli random variables, the sum of which is a binomial random variable.

Poisson-Characterized by a value lambda, equal to 1/mean. Poisson distribution is often used to characterize the number of events that occur per unit of time— for example, the average rate at which cars arrive at a toll plaza.

Patterned-Characterized by a lower and upper bound, a step, repetition rate for values, and repetition rate for the sequence.

Discrete-Characterized by a value and the associated probability range. The range must contain two columns: The left column contains values, and the right column contains probabilities associated with the value in that row. The sum of the probabilities must be 1.

Parameters-Enter values to characterize the distribution selected.

Random Seed-Enter an optional value from which to generate random numbers.

Output Range-Enter the reference for the upper-left cell of the output table. Excel automatically determines the size of the output area and displays a message if the output table will replace existing data.

New Worksheet Ply-Click to insert a new worksheet in the current workbook and paste the results starting at cell A1 of the new worksheet. To name the new worksheet, type a name in the box.

New Workbook-Click to create a new workbook and paste the results on a new worksheet in the new workbook.

II. Plotting graphs and obtaining trend line to find relations in input and out put.

One can plot various types of graphs using Chart Wizard function available in Excel Toolbar. After entering data one can click on chart wizard to select the type of graph to be plotted. Many graph patterns are available and it gives several options in each pattern.

This function can be used to plot graph for response (output) to standard (test) input that can be used for calculation of input value from the response (output).

Trendline: A graphic representation of trends in data series, such as a line sloping upward to represent increased response over a increase in input. Trendlines are used for the study of problems of prediction, also called regression analysis.

1. Enter data

2. Plot graph-Chart Wizard-select-XY scatter-get graph.

3. Right click on any point on graph to get Format Data Series, Click-Add trendline.

4. Select Type (usually linear)

5. Select Options- set intercept (if sure that intercept to pass 0 click or leave as it is), click on Display equation on chart and also Display R^2 value

R^2 *value* - Also known as the coefficient of determination. A number from 0 to 1 that reveals how closely the estimated values for the trendline correspond to actual data. A trendline is most reliable when its R-squared value is at or near 1. It can be seen in next figures that how changing in values of points far away from the central tendency to near central tendency increases the R^2 **value** towards unity.

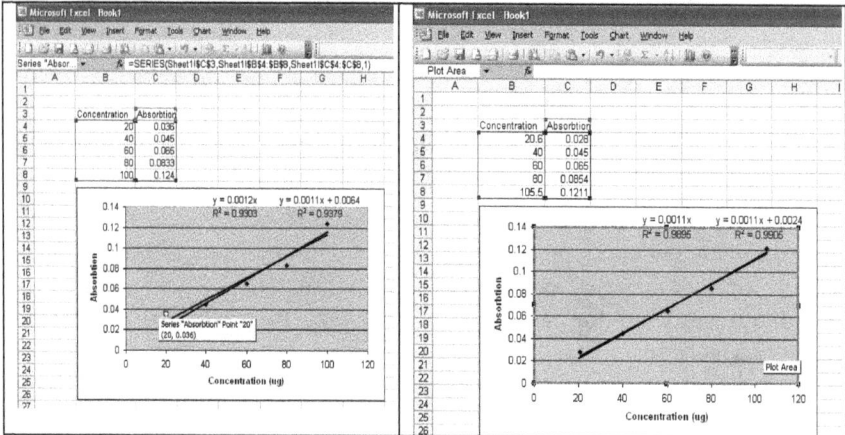

In above figures- as the points come near central tendency the R^2 **values** changed from 0.93 to .99.

Two equations for the line (slope of line) one for intercept passing through 0 (if it theoretically possible e.g. conc vs absorbtion) and second for intercept not passing through 0 (In cases like dose –response graphs)

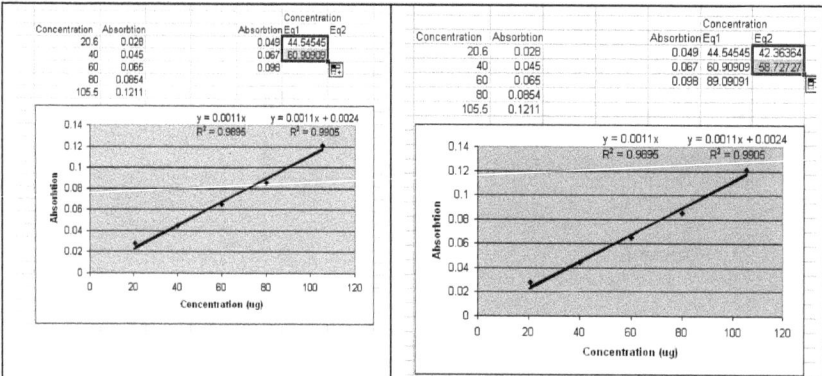

The equations obtained are used for calculation of input (Concentration of unknown) from the output information (response i.e Absorption). By entering formula one can get direct answer for every input.

If someone need to perform more complicated regression analysis (A form of statistical analysis used for forecasting. which estimates the relationship between variables so that a given variable can be predicted from one or more other variables), it can be performed using function available in analysis tool as mentioned above and shown below for descriptive statistics.

III.   Data Analysis to find descriptive statistics and ANOVA

Consider 4 experimental groups namely A, B, C and D are treated with different treatment. Each group is having 6 animals and we wish to find out the Mean, SEM or SD etc along with ANOVA, which will enable person to whether the results of different groups are significantly different or not.

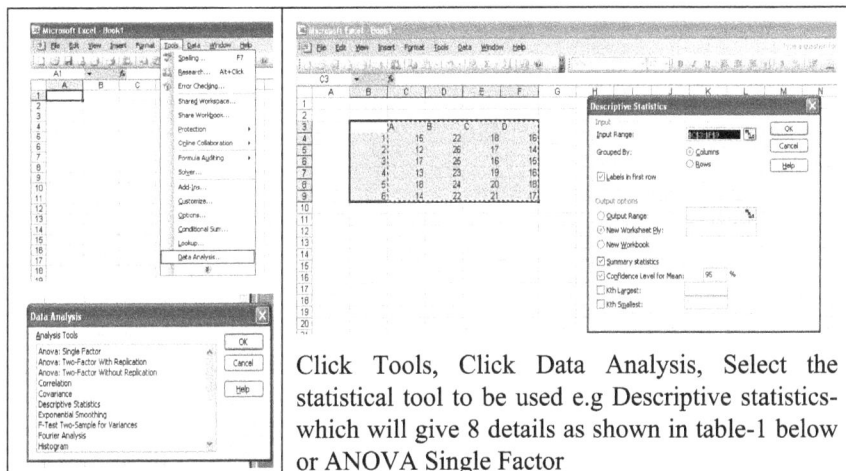

Click Tools, Click Data Analysis, Select the statistical tool to be used e.g Descriptive statistics-which will give 8 details as shown in table-1 below or ANOVA Single Factor

About the Anova: Single Factor dialog box

Input Range: Enter the cell reference for the range of data one want to analyze. The reference must consist of two or more adjacent ranges of data arranged in columns or rows.

Grouped By: To indicate whether the data in the input range is arranged in rows or in columns, click Rows or Columns.

Labels in First Row/Labels in First Column: If the first row of your input range contains labels, select the Labels in First Row check box. If the labels are in the first column of your input range, select the Labels in First Column check box. This check box is clear if your input range has no labels; Microsoft Excel generates appropriate data labels for the output table.

Alpha: Enter the level at which one want to evaluate critical values for the F statistic. The alpha level is a significance level related to the probability of having a type I error (rejecting a true hypothesis).

Output Range: Enter the reference for the upper-left cell of the output table. Excel automatically determines the size of the output area and displays a message if the output table will replace existing data or extend beyond the bounds of the worksheet.

New Worksheet Ply: Click to insert a new worksheet in the current workbook and paste the results starting at cell A1 of the new worksheet. To name the new worksheet, type a name in the box.

New Workbook: Click to create a new workbook and paste the results on a new worksheet in the new workbook.

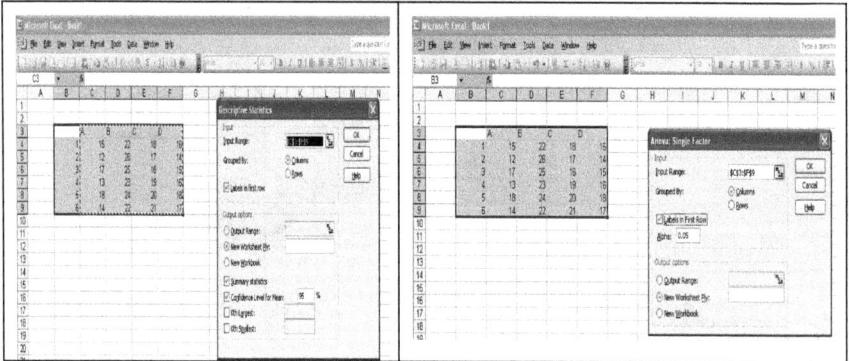

Table 11.1 showing the results after performing descriptive statistics application for the given data.

A		B		C		D	
Mean	14.83333	Mean	23.66667	Mean	18.5	Mean	16
Standard Error	0.945751	Standard Error	0.666667	Standard Error	0.763763	Standard Error	0.57735
Median	14.5	Median	23.5	Median	18.5	Median	16
Mode	#N/A	Mode	22	Mode	#N/A	Mode	16
Standard Deviation	2.316607	Standard Deviation	1.632993	Standard Deviation	1.870829	Standard Deviation	1.414214
Sample Variance	5.366667	Sample Variance	2.666667	Sample Variance	3.5	Sample Variance	2
Kurtosis	-1.41777	Kurtosis	-1.48125	Kurtosis	-1.2	Kurtosis	-0.3
Skewness	0.300289	Skewness	0.382733	Skewness	0	Skewness	5E-17
Range	6	Range	4	Range	5	Range	4
Minimum	12	Minimum	22	Minimum	16	Minimum	14
Maximum	18	Maximum	26	Maximum	21	Maximum	18
Sum	89	Sum	142	Sum	111	Sum	96
Count	6	Count	6	Count	6	Count	6
Confidence Level(95.0%)	2.43113	Confidence Level(95.0%)	1.713721	Confidence Level(95.0%)	1.963314	Confidence Level(95.0%)	1.484126

Anova: Single Factor					
SUMMARY					
Groups	Count	Sum	Average	Variance	
A	6	89	14.83333	5.366667	
B	6	142	23.66667	2.666667	
C	6	111	18.5	3.5	
D	6	96	16	2	
ANOVA					
Source of Variation	SS	df	MS	F	P-value	F crit
Between Groups	276.8333	3	92.27778	27.27422	2.87E-07	3.098391
Within Groups	67.66667	20	3.383333			
Total	344.5	23			

P value less than 0.05 indicates that the difference in the results produced by various groups differs significantly meaning that the differences are NOT by Chance but truly due the difference in activity of different agent.

Standard deviation (SD)

The standard deviation (SD) quantifies variability or scatter. If the data follow a bell shaped Gaussian distribution, then 68% of the values lie within one SD of the mean (on either side) and 95% of the values lie within two SD of the mean. The SD is expressed in the same units of the given data.

The standard deviation computed this way (with a denominator of N-1) is called the sample SD, in contrast to the population SD which would have a denominator of N. Why is the denominator N-1 rather than N? In the numerator, one computes the difference between each value and the mean of those values. No one knows the true mean of the population; all any one knows is the mean of the given sample. Except for the rare cases where the sample mean happens to equal the population mean, the data will be closer to the sample mean than it will be to the population mean. This means that the numerator will be too small. So the denominator is reduced as well. It is reduced to N-1 because that is the number of degrees of freedom in the given data. When computing the SD of a list of values, one can calculate the last value from N-1 of the values, so statisticians say there are N-1 degrees of freedom.

Standard error of the mean (SEM)

The standard error of the mean (SEM) quantifies the precision of the mean. It is a measure of how far the given sample mean is likely to be from the true population mean.

With large samples, the SEM is always small. By itself, the SEM is difficult to interpret. It is easier to interpret the 95% confidence interval, which is calculated from the SEM.

The difference between the SD and SEM

It is easy to be confused about the difference between the standard deviation (SD) and the standard error of the mean (SEM).

The SD quantifies scatter — how much the values vary from one another.

The SEM quantifies how accurately one know the true mean of the population. The SEM gets smaller as the given samples get larger. This makes sense, because the mean of a large sample is likely to be closer to the true population mean than is the mean of a small sample.

The SD does not change predictably as one acquire more data. The SD quantifies the scatter of the data, and increasing the size of the sample does not change the scatter. The SD might go up, or it might go down; one can't predict. On average, the SD will stay the same as sample size gets larger.

If the scatter is caused by biological variability, some one probably will want to show the variation. In this case, report the SD rather than the SEM. If some one is using an in vitro system with no biological variability, the scatter can only result from experimental imprecision. In this case, person may not want to show the scatter, but instead show how well one have assessed the mean. Report the mean and SEM, or the mean with 95% confidence interval.

One should choose to show the SD or SEM based on the source of the variability and the point of the experiment. In fact, many scientists choose the SEM simply because it is smaller so creates shorter error bars.

95% confidence interval (CI)

Like the SEM, the confidence interval also quantifies the precision of the mean. The mean one calculates from the given sample of data points depends on which values one happened to sample. Therefore, the mean one calculates is unlikely to equal the overall population mean exactly. The size of the likely discrepancy depends on the variability of the values (expressed as the SD) and the sample size. Combine those together to calculate a 95% confidence interval (95% CI), which is a range of values. One can be 95% sure that this interval contains the true population mean. More precisely, if one generate many 95% CIs from many data sets, he expect the CI to include the true population mean in 95% of the cases and not to include the true mean value in the other 5% of the cases. Since one doesn't know the population mean, he will never know when this happens.

The confidence interval extends in each direction by a distance calculated from the standard error of the mean multiplied by a critical value from the t distribution. This value depends on the degree of confidence one want (traditionally 95%, but it is possible to calculate intervals for any degree of confidence) and on the number of degrees of freedom in this experiment (N-1). With large samples, this multiplier equals 1.96. With smaller samples, the multiplier is larger.

Coefficient of variation (CV)

The coefficient of variation (CV), also known as "relative variability", equals the standard deviation divided by the mean (expressed as a percent). Because it is a unitless ratio, one can compare the CV of variables expressed in different units. It only makes sense to report CV for a variable, such as mass or enzyme activity, where "0.0" is defined to really mean zero. A weight of zero means no weight. An enzyme activity of zero means no enzyme activity. In contrast, a temperature of "0.0" does not mean zero temperature (unless measured in degrees Kelvin). Don't calculate CV for variables, such as temperature, where the definition of zero is arbitrary.

It never makes sense to calculate the CV of a variable expressed as a logarithm because the definition of zero is arbitrary. The logarithm of 1 equals 0, so the log will equal zero whenever the actual value equals 1. By changing units, one'll redefine zero, so redefine the CV. The CV of a logarithm is, therefore, meaningless.

Quartiles and range

Quartiles divide the data into four groups, each containing an equal number of values. Quartiles are divided by the 25th percentile, 50th percentile, and 75th percentile. One quarter of the values are less than or equal to the 25th percentile. Three quarters of the values are less than or equal to the 75 th percentile. The median is the 50th percentile.

Prism computes percentile values by first computing $P*(N+1)/100$, where P is 25, 50, or 75 and N is the number of values in the data set. The result is the rank that corresponds to the percentile value. If there are 68 values, the 25th percentile corresponds to a rank equal to $25*(68+1)/100 =17.25$, so the 25th percentile lies between the value of the 17th and 18th value (when ranked from low to high). Prism computes the 25th percentile as the average of those two values.

While there is no ambiguity about how to calculate the median, there are several ways to compute the 25th and 75th percentiles. Prism uses what is probably the most commonly used method. With large data sets, all the methods give similar results. With small data sets, the results can vary quite a bit.

Geometric mean

The geometric mean is the antilog of the mean of the logarithms of the values. This is the same as taking the Nth root (where N is the number of points) of the product of all N values. It is less affected by outliers than the mean. Prism also reports the 95% confidence interval of the geometric mean.

Skewness and kurtosis

Skewness quantifies the asymmetry of a distribution. A symmetrical distribution has a skewness of zero. An asymmetrical distribution with a long tail to the right (higher values) has a positive skew. An asymmetrical distribution with a long tail to the left (lower values) has a negative skew.

Kurtosis quantifies how closely the shape of a distribution follows the usual Gaussian shape. A Gaussian distribution, by definition, has a kurtosis of 0. A distribution with more values in the center, and less in the tails, has a negative kurtosis. A distribution with fewer values in the center and more in the tail has a positive kurtosis.

Appendix 1

CPCSEA Registration Requirements

1. Registration details of the organization

2. Details of trained staff available for animal experiments (Person/s in charge of animal house)

3. Resume of each individual appointed by the organization on IAEC with their letter of consent stating that they are aware about duties and obligations as per Breeding of and Experimentation on Animals (CPCSEA) Rules 1998.

4. Proceedings of last IAEC meeting with resolutions to request CPCSEA for registration

5. Layout plan for animal house facilities

6. Details about animal to be used for experiments (Species/strain/sex/age/number)

7. Facilities available for conduction of experiments with information about condition of animals before and after experiments

8. Name and address of establishment from where animals can be received

9. Mode of transport of animals

10. Protocol (Part A and B) filled separately s.

11. If imported animals detailed protocol to justify the need of imported animals

12. One self addressed stamped post-card

Appendix 2

Part B to be Submitted to IAEC for Approval of Protocol for Animal Experimentation.

NAME of INSTITUTE/ORGANIZATION

Protocol form for research proposals to be submitted to the Institutional Animal Ethics Committee, for new experiments or extensions of ongoing experiments using animals other than non-human primates (PART B).

1. **Project title**:-

2. **Chief Investigator-**

    (a) Name

    (b) Designation

    (c) Dept/Div/Lab

    (d) Telephone number

3. **List of names of all individuals authorized to conduct procedures under this proposal**:-

4. **Funding Source**:-

5. **Duration of the project**:-.

    (a) Number of months

    (b) Date of initiation

    (c) Date of completion

6. **If date by which approval is needed is less than six weeks from date of submission, justification for the same**:-

7. **Study Objectives, the aims of study (and why they are important) to be explained briefly using non-technical terms as far as possible)**:-

8. **Animals required**

    (a) Species:-

    (b) Age/Weight/Size:-

    (c) Gender:-

    (d) Numbers to be used (Year-wise break-ups and total figures needed to be given):-

    (e) Numbers of days each animal will be housed :-

9. **Rationale for animal usage: -** (details to be given in 5-6 lines for each question)

    (a) Why is animal usage necessary for these studies?

    (b) Why are the particular species selected required?

    (c) Why are the estimated number of animals essential?

    (d) Similar experiments conducted in the past. If so, the number of animals used and results obtained in brief.

    (e) If yes, why new experiment is required?

    (f) Have similar experiment(s) been made by any other organization/agency? If so, their results in your knowledge.

10. **Description of   procedures to be used**: - (details to be given in 5-6 lines)

11. **Does the protocol prohibit use of anaesthetic or analgesic for the conduct of painful procedures (any which cause more pain than that associated with routine injection, or blood withdrawal)? If yes, explanation and justification**

12. **Will survival surgery be done?** If yes, the following to be described

    (a) List and description of all such surgical procedures (including methods of asepsis)

    (b) Names, qualifications and experience levels of operators

    (c) Description of post-operative care

    (d) Justification if major survival surgery is to be performed more than once on a single individual animal

13. **Methods of disposal post-experimentation:-**

    Rehabilitation/Euthanasia (In case of euthanasia, justification for not undertaking rehabilitation and drug dosage and route for anaesthesia, where appropriate, as well as methods of carcass disposal)

14. **Animal transportation methods if extra-institutional transport is envisaged:-**

15. **Use of hazardous agents** (Use of recombinant DNA-based agents or potential human pathogens requires documented approval of the Institutional Biosafety Committee (IBC).For each category, the agents and the biosafety level required, appropriate therapeutic measures and the mode of disposal of contaminated food animal wastes and carcasses must be identified).

   (a)   Radionuclides

   (b)   Biological Agents

   (c)   Hazardous chemicals or drugs

   (d)   Recombinant DNA

   (e)   Any other (give name)

Copy of IBC approval to be attached in case hazardous agents are used

Investigator's declaration

1. I certify that I have determined that the research proposal herein is not unnecessarily duplicative of previously reported research

2. I certify that all individuals working on this proposal, and experimenting on the animals, have been trained in animal handling procedures.

3. For procedures listed under item 11, I certify that I have reviewed the pertinent scientific literature and have found no valid alternative to any procedure described herein which may cause less pain or distress.

4. I will obtain approval from the IAEC/CPCSEA before initiating any significant changes in this study.

5. Certified that performance of experiment will be initiated only upon review and approval of scientific intent by appropriate expert body [Institutional Scientific Advisory Committee/funding agency/other body (to be named)].

6. Institutional Biosafety Committee's (IBC) certification of review and concurrence will be taken (Required for studies utilizing DNA agents of human pathogens.

7. I shall maintain all the records as per format (Form D).

Signature   Date:

                                        Name of Investigator

(for IAEC/CPCSEA usage)

Proposal number:-

Date first received:-

Date received after modification (if any):-

Date received after second modification (if any):-

Approval Date: _

Expiry Date:-

Names of IAEC Chairperson /CPCSEA Nominee:-

Signatures   Chairperson

CPCSEA Nominee

Date

Appendix 3

Breeding of and Experiments on Animals (Control and Supervision) Rules, 1998 MINISTRY OF SOCIAL JUSTICE & EMPOWERMENT NOTIFICATION

New Delhi, the 15th December, 1998

S.O. 1074.—Whereas the draft Breeding of and Experiments on Animals (Control and Supervision) Rules, 1998 were published, as required by sub section (1) of Section 17 of, the Prevention of Cruelty to Animals Act, 1960 (59 of 1960) under the notification of the Government of India, Ministry of environment and Forests number S.O. 789(E) dated, the e September, 1998 in the Gazette of India, Extraordinary , Part II, section 31 Sub-section (ii) inviting objections and suggestion from all the persons likely to be affected thereby, before the expiry of the period of thirty days from the date on which copies of the Gazette, containing the said notification are made available to the public; And, whereas the said Gazette was made available to the public on 8th September, 1998. And whereas the objections/suggestions received in respect of the said draft rules, have been duly considered-by the Committee for control and supervision of experiments on animals;

Now, therefore, in exercise of the powers conferred by sub-section (1) (1A) and (2) of section 17 of the Prevention of Cruelty to Animals Act, 196 (59 of 1960), the Committee for control and supervision of experiments on animals hereby makes the following rules, namely:

1. **Short Title and commencement.** 1. These rules may be called the Breeding of and Experiments on Animals (Control and Supervision) Rules, 1998. 2. They shall come into force on the date of their publication in the Official Gazette.

2. **Definitions.** - In these rules, unless the context otherwise requires -

    (a) "Act" means the Prevention of Cruelty to Animals Act, 1960 (59 of 1960);

(b) "breeder" means a person including an institution, which breeds animals for the purpose of transfer to other authorised institution for performing experiments;

(c) "Committee" means the Committee under section 15 of the Act for control and supervision of experiments on animals;

(d) "establishment means any individual, company, firm, corporation, institution other than schools up to higher secondary level, which performs experiments on animals;

(e) "experiment" means any programme/project involving experiments on an animal /animals for the purpose of advancement by new discovery of physiological knowledge which will be useful for saving or prolonging life or alleviating suffering or for combating any disease whether on human beings or animals; (Amendment[1]- and giving significant gains in the well being of the people of country)

(f) "Institutional Animals Ethics Committee" means a body comprising of a group of persons recognised and registered by the Committee for the purpose of control and supervision of experiments on animal performed in an establishment which is constituted and operated in accordance with procedures specified for the purpose by the Committee;

(g) "contract Research" means any research undertaken by an individual, company, firm, corporation or institution on behalf of a foreign individual, company, firm, corporation or institution for any consideration;

(h) "collaborative research" means any research undertaken between two or more research institutions on an equal footing which does not involve any financial or monetary considerations and is undertaken solely for the purpose of advancement of scientific research and human welfare;

(i) "specified format" means the form specified for the purpose by the Committee from time to time.

3. Breading of animals

(a) No establishment shall carry on the business of breeding of animals or trade of animals for the purpose of experiments unless it is registered.

---

[1] Amendment / amended- Amendments circulated with the CPCSEA guidelines on regulation of Scientific Experiments on Animals by Ministry of Environment and Forest (animal Welfare Division), Govt. of India. June 2007

(b) Every breeder/establishment carrying on the business of breeding animals or trade of animals for the purpose of experiments, shall, apply for registration within sixty days from the date of commencement of these rules and, stop breeding of animals if registration is subsequently refused to it by the Committee.

4. Registration of establishments

(a) No establishment shall perform any experiment on animals unless it is registered.

(b) Every establishment performing experiments on animals, shall, apply for registration within sixty days from the date of commencement of these rules and, stop performing experiments on animals if registration is subsequently refused to it by the Committee.

5. Application for registration

(a) The application for registration by a breeder under sub-rule (b) of rule 3 and an establishment under sub-rule (b) of rule 4 shall be made in the specified format to the Member- Secretary or any other officer authorised in this regard by the Committee.

(b) The Member-Secretary or the authorised officer of the Committee, may for deciding the issue of registration, ask for information relating to premises where the experiments are to be conducted, animal housing facilities, details of breeding of animals and its trade, other infrastructure including availability of manpower trained in handling animals and for verification of facts mentioned in the application for registration, and if satisfied, shall register such establishment or the breeder.

(c) A breeder or the establishment on registration for the purpose of performing experiments on animals shall comply with the conditions as may be specified, at the time of registration, by the Member-Secretary of the Committee or any officer authorised in this regard by the Committee.

6. Details of the experiments conducted

(a) Every registered establishment shall maintain a register as per the specified format and keep complete particulars about the kind of animal to be used for conducting any experiment, the health of the animal, the nature of experiment to be performed, and the reasons necessitating the performance of such an experiment on particular species.

(b)   The Member-Secretary or the officer authorised by the Committee in this behalf may examine the register so maintained, and if, he is not satisfied irrespective -of the -opportunity given for improvement, he may bring the same to the notice of the Committee seeking directions in this regard.

7. **Stocking of animals:** The animals shall be stocked by the breeder and the establishment in the following manner:-

(a)   animal houses shall be located in a quiet atmosphere undisturbed by traffic, and the premises kept tidy, hygienic and the animals protected from drought and extremes of weather;

(b)   animal cages for small animals and stables for large animals shall be such that animals can live in comfort and overcrowding is avoided;

(c)   where standards have been laid down by the Indian Standards Institution, the cages, the stable, as the case may be, shall conform to those standards;

(d)   animals attendants must be suitably trained and experienced in the duties allotted to them,

(e)   animals shall be looked after, before and after the experiments by a trained and experienced attendant;

(f)   there-shall be satisfactory arrangement for looking after the animals during off hours and on holidays,

8. **Permission of the Committee required for conducting experiments:**

(a)   Every registered establishment before acquiring an animal or conducting any experiment on an animal/animals shall apply for permission of the Committee or the Institutional Animals Ethics Committee recognised for the purpose by the Committee along with the details contained in the specified format to the Member Secretary of the Committee or the Institutional Animals Ethics Committee, as the case may be.

(b)   The Member Secretary of the Committee or the Institutional Animals Ethics Committee, shall cause the application for permission to be brought before the Committee/Institutional Animals Ethics Committee as the case may be, and the Committee/ Institutional Animals Ethics Committee after scrutiny of the application, if satisfied, may grant permission to the establishment stating the name of the species and the number of animals that can be acquired for carrying out the experiments.

(c)   The Committee or Institutional Animals Ethics Committee, as the case may be, may, while granting permission for conducting experiments on animals, put conditions as it may deem fit to ensure that animals are not subjected to unnecessary pain or suffering before, during or after the performance of experiments on them.

(d) The Committee may require the establishments and Institutional Animals Ethics Committees and persons carrying on experiments on animals to forward to the Committee such information as it may require, on completion of experiments for which the permission has been granted.

9. **Performance of experiments:** In conducting experiments on animals, regard shall be had to the following conditions, namely:

(a) experiments shall be performed in every case by or under the supervision of a person duly qualified in that behalf, that is, Degree or Diploma holders in Veterinary Science or Medicine or Laboratory Animal Science of a University or an Institution recognised by the Government for the purpose and under the responsibility of the person performing the experiment;

(b) experiments shall be performed with due care and humanity;

(bb) amended- The preference to be accorded to the use of minimum number of animals, lowest in the phylogenetic scale, which provide for statistically valid results at 95% degree of confidence. Use of replacement/alternatives is encouraged and sound justification is required in case alternatives to use animals are not used, when available.

(c) animals intended for the performance of experiments are properly looked both before and after experiments;

(cc) amended- The personnel using animals in experiment responsible for their welfare after use in experimentation, including aftercare and rehabilitation to be made part of the research costs, as a lump sum provision based on the statistically expected life span of the animals. Rehabilitation may be undertaken by the establishment or by a duly licensed and authorized animal welfare organization.

(d) experiments involving operative procedure more severe than simple inoculation or superficial venesection shall be performed under the influence of anaesthetic to prevent the animal feeling pain and it shall remain so throughout the experiment. Anaesthesia shall be administered by a Veterinary Surgeon trained in methods of anaesthesia or a Scientist/technician so trained for this purpose and who shall remain present near the animal till the completion of the experiment;

(e) animals which in the course of experiments under the influence of anaesthetic are so injured that their recovery would involve pain or suffering shall be destroyed humanely while still under the influence of anaesthesia;

(f)   when there is reason to believe that an animal is suffering abnormal or severe pain at any stage of a continuing experiment, it shall be painlessly destroyed at that stage without proceeding with the experiment;

(ff) amended-The specific parameters, which are to be adopted when considering euthanisation of any animal used in scientific experiments. These include impairment of the natural function of the animal including independent locomotion, when the animal faces recurring pain suffering, and when the non termination of the life of experimental animal would be life threatening to humans or other animals

(g)   the experiment shall not be performed for the purpose of attaining or retaining manual skill except in schools, colleges and recognised training institutions;

(h)   experiments shall not be performed by way of an illustration;

(i)   experiments shall not be performed as a public demonstration;

(j)   the substance known as Urari or Curari or any such paralysing shall not be used or administered for the purpose of any experiment except in conjunction with anaesthetic of sufficient depth to produce loss of consciousness;

(k)   no experiment the result of which is already conclusively known, shall be repeated without previous justification;

(l)   there shall not be applied to the eye of an animal by way of experiment any chemical substance for the purpose of absorption through the conjunctival membrane or through the cornea calculated to only give pain;

(m) dogs held for experimental purposes shall not be debarked.

(n)   where experiments are performed in any institution, the responsibility therefore is placed on the person in charge of the institution and in cases where experiments are performed outside an institution by an individual qualified in that behalf, the-experiments, are performed on his responsibility.

10. Transfer and acquisition of animals for experiment:

(a)   A breeder shall not transfer any animal by sale or otherwise to an establishment which is not registered under these' rules.

(b)   An establishment shall not acquire any animal by sale or otherwise except from a registered breeder/establishment. Amended-The establishment will be allowed to procure animals from any other legal sources in case of non-availability with the registered breeders, with suitable documentation to legality of the procurement process.

(c) Every establishment after acquisition of an animal or animals shall not transfer such animal or animals by sale or otherwise to any other establishment or person except to a registered breeder/establishment.

(d) The animals used for experimentation in a production/ breed improvement programme may be given out by the breeder' institution for domestic use.

(e) No animal shall be imported by a breeder or an establishment which is available in the country. Amended-The establishment will be allowed to import genetically defined animals with the permission of DGFT, in case such animals are available with registered breeders or other legal sources within the country. The condition of non-availability will not apply to genetically defined or laboratory bred rats and mice.

(f) A breeder or establishment shall comply, with the directions given by the Committee for the purpose of controlling and supervising experiments on animals.

11.   Records

(a) Every, establishment/Institutional Animals Ethics Committee shall maintain a record of the animals under its control and custody in the specified format.

(b) Every establishment/Institutional Animals Ethics Committee shall furnish such information, as the Committee may from time to time require in the specified format.

(c) All laboratories shall inform the exact number/ species of animals to the Member Secretary or any officer authorised in this regard by the Committee as per the specified format.

12.   Contract animal experiments: No establishment shall contract or undertake to perform contract research or experiments on contract basis on behalf of any other establishment or research or educational Institution, This shall not apply to collaborative research between academic institutions. Amended- The establishment will be allowed to undertake contract research as per the provisions of PCA Act 1960 and the rules made there under.

13.   Composition of Institutional Animals Ethics Committee: Every Institutional Animals Ethics committee shall include a biological scientist, two scientists from different biological disciplines, a veterinarian involved in the care of animal, the scientist in charge of animals facility of the establishment concerned, a scientist from, outside the institute, a non scientific socially aware member and a representative or nominee of the specialist may be co-opted while reviewing special project using hazardous agents such as radio-active substance and deadly micro organisms.

14. Power to suspend or revolve registration:

(a) If the Committee is satisfied, on the report of the Member-Secretary of the authorised officer of the Committee made to it as a result of any inspection or information received otherwise that the rules made by it are not being complied with by any establishment or breeder or an Institutional Animals Ethics Committee, the Committee may, after giving a reasonable opportunity to the establishment or breeder or Institutional Animals Ethics Committee of being heard in the matter, revoke the registration of such establishment or breeder or Institutional Animals Ethics Committee either for a specified period or indefinitely, or may allow the establishment of- breeder or Institutional Animals Ethics Committee to carry on subject to such special conditions as the Committee may impose.

(b) The Committee may, pending the final determination, if, it is of the opinion that an establishment or breeder has prima facie failed to comply with the provisions of these Riles, suspend the registration of such establishment or the breeder.

(c) The Committee may in the event of revocation or suspension of registration of an establishment or breeder, issue such directions as it, deems fit for the care and protection of the animals which are under the custody or control of such establishment or the breeder.

(d) That in the event of suspension or revocation of a license, such establishment or breeder shall forthwith on the communication of the order cease to perform any experiment on, any animal or acquire or transfer any animal.

Amended- The CPCSEA shall take action against an establishment or breeder, based on the report of the member Secretary or authorized officer, regarding any violations of the rules, or of directions of the Committee. In case of a major violation, CPCSEA may by written orders, suspend or revoke the registration of the establishment and /r order closure of animal house facility, after giving the establishment or breeder an opportunity of being heard in the matter.

{F. No. 7-5/98-AW]

ASHOK PAL SINGH, Member Secretary

Committee for the Purpose of Control &

Supervision of Experiments on Animals

Bibliography

Brunton LL, Editor. Goodman. Gilman's The Pharmacological Basis of Therapeutics. Eleventh Edition. McGraw-Hill Medical Publishing Division.

CPCSEA guidelines as available from website of CPCSEA.

Gosh MN. Fundamentals of Experimental Pharmacology. Third Edition (2005). Hilton and Company, Kolkata.

Goyal RK. Practicals in Pharmacology. Eighth Edition (2008-09). BS Shah Prakashan, Ahmedabad.

Rang HP, Dale MM, Ritter JM and Flower RJ. Rang and Dales Pharmacology. Sixth Edition (2008). Churchil LivingStone, Sinagpore.

UH Handbook of Experimental Animals.

Vogel H.G. Editor.Drug Discovery and Evaluation Pharmacological Assays. Second Edition (2002). Springer Verlag. Berlin

Websites

www.nc3rs.org.uk

www.labanimals.no

http://www.vetmed.ucdavis.edu/

http://www.wisc.edu/

http://dels.nas.edu/

http://research.uiowa.edu/

http://www.pdg.cnb.uam.es/cursos/Barcelona2002/pages/Farmac

http://www.nal.usda.gov/awic/pubs/

JOURNAL

EFPIA/ECVAM paper on good practice in administration of substances and removal of blood, J Appl Toxicol 21 15-23, 2001.

www.ingramcontent.com/pod-product-compliance
Lightning Source LLC
Chambersburg PA
CBHW050646190326
41458CB00008B/2438